# Clinical Handbook
# of Psychotropic Drugs

**second revised edition**

Kalyna Z. Bezchlibnyk-Butler, BScPhm
*Principal Editor*

J. Joel Jeffries, MB, FRCP(C)
*Co-Editor*

Sandra B. Bredin, BScPhm
Suvndram Naidoo, BScPhm
Carol E. Friesen, BScPhm
*Contributing Editors*

*Clarke Institute of Psychiatry, Toronto, Canada*

**Hogrefe & Huber Publishers**

**Toronto • Lewiston, NY • Bern • Göttingen • Stuttgart**

**Library of Congress Cataloging-in-Publication Data**
The first edition of this book was published under:
Clinical handbook of psychotropic drugs / Kalyna Z. Bezchlibnyk-Butler,
principal editor, J. Joel Jeffries, co-editor ; Sandra B.
Bredin, Suvndram Naidoo, Carol E. Friesen, contributing editors.
      p.      cm
  Bibliography:  p.
  ISBN 0-920887-38-4
    1.   Psychotropic drugs--Handbooks, manuals, etc.    I.  Bezchlibyk-
Butler, Kalyna Z., 1947-       II. Jeffries, J. Joel, 1929-    .
RM315.C547       1989               88-21704
615'.788--dc19                      CIP


**Canadian Cataloguing in Publication Data**

Main entry under title:

Clinical handbook of psychotropic drugs
2nd rev. ed.
Includes bibliographical references

ISBN 0-920887-86-4

1. Psychotropic drugs - Handbooks, manuals, etc.
I. Bezchlibnyk-Butler, Kalyna Z., 1947- .
II. Jeffries, J. Joel, 1939-      .

RM315.C55        1990     615'.788     C89-095274-4

**Copyright ©1990 by Hans Huber Publishers, Inc.**

Printed in Canada

**ISBN 0-920887-86-4**     **Hans Huber Publishers  Toronto • Lewiston, NY**
**ISBN 3-456-81866-1**     **Hans Huber Publishers  Bern • Stuttgart**

# TABLE OF CONTENTS

# ANTIDEPRESSANTS

**CLASSES**

**Cyclic Antidepressants:** Tricyclic, Dibenzoxazepine, Tetracyclic, Triazolopyridine, Monocyclic, Bicyclic

**Monoamine Oxidase Inhibitors (MAOIs)**

**INDICATIONS**

- Treatment of major depressions; tricyclics and related groups are less effective for reactive or mild depressions
- Treatment and prophylaxis of recurrent depressions, as in unipolar affective disorder
- Panic disorder prophylaxis
- Phobic disorders
- Obsessive-compulsive disorder (clomipramine)
- Treatment of enuresis in children and adolescents (imipramine, other tricyclics)
- Others include: migraine headache, pain, ulcers

**GENERAL COMMENTS**

- Antidepressants reduce the degree of depression and usually increase psychomotor activity before affecting the depression; as energy increases, the risk of suicide may persist — this must be watched for at all times
- If tricyclics (or related drugs) and MAO inhibitors are to be used together, neither should be administered parenterally; both can be started together or the MAO inhibitor can be initiated *after* the tricyclic; patients should be carefully monitored for hypertension and other side effects
- Maximum antidepressant effects may not be apparent for 2 or more weeks

**THERAPEUTIC EFFECTS**

- Elevation of mood, improved appetite and sleep patterns, increased physical activity, improved mental functioning, decreased feelings of guilt, worthlessness, inadequacy and ambivalence, decrease in delusional preoccupation
- Combined therapy with lithium may increase antidepressant effect

**DEXAMETHASONE SUPPRESSION TEST (DST)**

- When a healthy person receives dexamethasone, cortisol levels in the blood are generally suppressed over 24 hours, while approximately 50-70% of patients with clinically diagnosed major depression fail to suppress cortisol following dexamethasone administration

**DST Protocol**

1) Administer 1 mg dexamethasone orally at 2300 hrs on Day 1
2) The following day, draw venous blood for a cortisol assay at 1530 and 2200 hrs

- The test is considered positive if either of the two plasma cortisol levels is 140 nmol/L or higher
- From a clinical standpoint, a negative DST does not rule out a valid diagnosis of depression

# Cyclic Antidepressants

**DOSES**

- See page 10

**PHARMACOLOGY**

- Exact mechanism of action unknown; equilibrate the effects of biogenic amines through various mechanisms
- The action in the treatment of enuresis may involve inhibition of urination due to the anticholinergic effect and CNS stimulation, resulting in easier arousal by the stimulus of a full bladder

**PHARMACOKINETICS**

- Completely absorbed from the gastrointestinal tract; large percentage metabolized by firstpass effect
- Highly lipophilic; concentrated primarily in myocardial and cerebral tissue
- Highly bound to plasma protein
- Metabolized primarily by the liver
- Elimination half-life approximately 24 hrs (protriptyline = 78 hrs, trazodone = 8 hrs, fluoxetine = 96 hrs)

**DOSING ROUTE**

- Usual route of administration is oral - I. M. injection has no advantage except with patients unwilling or unable to receive drug orally
- There is a wide patient variation in dosage requirements (partly dependent on plasma levels)
- I. V. clomipramine up to 300 mg daily for treatment of obsessive compulsive disorder

**ONSET AND DURATION OF ACTION**

- Sedative effects are seen within a few hours of oral administration, with lessened sleep disturbances after a few days
- Therapeutic effect is seen after 7-28 days
- Tricyclics and related drugs are long-acting; they may be given in a single daily dose, usually at bedtime

**ADVERSE EFFECTS**

- See accompanying charts (pp. 11 and 12) for incidence of adverse effects

**1. Anticholinergic Effects**

- A result of antagonism at muscarinic receptors
- Occur frequently, especially in elderly patients
- Dry mucous membranes [Management: sugar-free gum and candy, oral lubricants (e.g., MoiStir, OraCare D, etc.), pilocarpine mouthwash (4 drops 4% solution to 12 drops water swished in mouth and spat out)]
- Blurred vision [Management: pilocarpine 1% eye drops]
- Dry eyes; may be of particular difficulty in the elderly or those wearing contact lenses [Management: artificial tears, but employ caution with patients wearing soft contact lenses; these patients should have their dry eyes managed with their usual wetting solutions or comfort drops]
- Constipation (frequent in children on therapy for enuresis) [Management: increase bulk and fluid intake, fecal softener, bulk laxative]
- Urinary retention, delayed micturition [Management: bethanechol]
- Sweating [Management: daily showering, talcum powder]

*Continued*

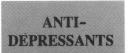

**ANTI-DEPRESSANTS**

# Cyclic Antidepressants (cont'd)

*Adverse effects (cont'd )*

**2. CNS Effects**

- A result of antagonism at histamine $H_1$-receptors and $\alpha_1$-adrenoreceptors
- Occur frequently
- Drowsiness (most common adverse effect) [Management: prescribe bulk of dose at bedtime]
- Weakness, lethargy, fatigue
- Conversely, excitement, nightmares, agitation, restlessness and insomnia have occurred; vivid dreaming can occur, especially if all the medication is given at bedtime
- Confusion, disturbed concentration, disorientation, delusions and hallucinations (more common in elderly)
- Precipitation of hypomania or mania, panic reactions, anxiety or euphoria may occur
- Seizures (more common in children)
- Children being treated for enuresis may experience drowsiness, anxiety, emotional instability, nervousness and sleep disorders
- Weight gain

**3. Neurological Effects**

- Fine tremor
- Akathisia (rare)
- Tardive dyskinesia (reported primarily with amoxapine, but also seen on rare occasions with other antidepressants)

**4. Cardiovascular Effects**

- A result of antagonism at $\alpha_1$-adrenoreceptors and inhibition of 5-HT uptake
- More common in elderly
- Tachycardia
- Orthostatic hypotension [Management: sodium chloride tablets, caffeine]
- Arrhythmias, syncope, thrombosis, thrombophlebitis, stroke, and congestive heart failure have been reported on occasion

**5. G.I. Effects**

- A result of inhibition of 5-HT uptake
- Anorexia, nausea, vomiting, diarrhea
- Peculiar taste, "black tongue," glossitis

**6. Endocrine**

- Increased or decreased libido, impotence [Management: bethanechol]
- Testicular swelling, breast engorgement, and breast tissue enlargement in males and females
- Anorgasmia in females [Management: cyproheptadine]
- Increase or decrease in blood sugar levels

**7. Allergic Reactions**

- Rare
- Jaundice, hepatitis, rash, urticaria, pruritis, edema
- Photosensitivity

**WITHDRAWAL SYMPTOMS**

- Abrupt withdrawal from high doses may cause a syndrome consisting of akathisia, anxiety, chills, coryza, malaise, myalgia, headache, dizziness, nausea and/or vomiting

☞ **THEREFORE, THESE MEDICATIONS SHOULD BE WITHDRAWN GRADUALLY AFTER PROLONGED USE**

## PRECAUTIONS

- Use cautiously in patients in whom excess anticholinergic activity could be harmful, e.g., prostatic hypertrophy, urinary retention, narrow-angle glaucoma
- Use with caution in patients with respiratory difficulties, as antidepressants can dry up bronchial secretions and make breathing more difficult
- May lower the seizure threshold; therefore, administer cautiously to patients with a history of convulsive disorders, organic brain disease, or a predisposition to convulsions, e.g., alcohol withdrawal
- May impair the mental and physical ability to perform hazardous tasks (e.g., driving a car or operating machinery); will potentiate the effects of alcohol
- May induce manic reactions in up to 50% of patients with bipolar affective disorder
- May lead to increased cycling of bipolar affective disorder
- Combination of fluoxetine with other cyclic antidepressants can lead to increased plasma level of other antidepressant

## TOXICITY

- The therapeutic margin is close to the toxic dose (lethal dose is about 3 times the maximum therapeutic dose)
- Symptoms of toxicity are extensions of the common adverse effects: anticholinergic, CNS stimulation followed by CNS depression
- Cardiac irregularities occur and are most hazardous; QRS duration on the electrocardiogram reflects the severity of the overdose; if it equals or exceeds 0.10 seconds, it should be considered to be a danger sign

## Treatment

- Physical removal of drug from G.I. tract (emesis with Ipecac,* lavage)
- Activated charcoal (40-50 g initially, followed by 20-25 g) decreases tricyclic antidepressant absorption and lowers its blood level. (DO NOT GIVE CONCURRENTLY WITH IPECAC)
- Supportive treatment, with patient closely monitored in a hospital
- Physostigmine salicylate injection (Antilirium) 1 mg I.M. counteracts both the central and peripheral anticholinergic effects
- I.V. diazepam or I.V. lorazepam are the drugs of choice for convulsions

## NURSING IMPLICATIONS

- Psychotherapy and education are also important in the treatment of depression
- Monitor therapy by watching for adverse side effects, mood and activity level changes; observe and chart all changes; keep physician informed
- Be aware that the medication reduces the degree of depression and may increase psychomotor activity; this may create concern about behaviour
- Expect a lag time of 7 to 28 days before antidepressant effects will be noticed
- Check for constipation; increase fluids and increase bulk in diet to lessen constipation
- Check for urinary retention; if required the physician may order bethanechol orally or by s.c. injection
- Warn patient to avoid driving a car or operating hazardous machinery until response to drug has been determined
- Reassure patient that drowsiness and dizziness usually subside after first few weeks; if dizzy, patient should get up from lying or sitting position slowly, and dangle legs over edge of bed before getting up
- Caution patient that alcohol or other CNS depressants will cause an increase in sleepiness, dizziness, and lightheadedness
- Excessive use of caffeinated foods, drugs, or beverages may increase anxiety and agitation and confuse the diagnosis
- Expect a dry mouth; suggest frequent mouth rinsing with water, and sour or sugarless hard candy or gum
- Warn patient to avoid extreme heat and humidity as these drugs may affect the body's ability to regulate temperature; photosensitivity reactions may occur on rare occasions so sunscreen agents may be indicated
- Artificial tears may be useful for patients who complain of dry eyes (or wetting solutions for those wearing contact lenses)

*Tincture of Ipecac: Emetic dose: 5-20 ml with plenty of water. Repeat if necessary in 1/2 hour. ☞ **DO NOT GIVE** to patients in shock, coma, or those who have ingested corrosive substances.

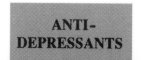

**ANTI-DEPRESSANTS**

# Cyclic Antidepressants (cont'd)

**USE IN PREGNANCY**

- Equivocal data indicate possible teratogenic effects, and therefore suggest avoiding antidepressants primarily in the first trimester

**Breast Milk**

- Antidepressants are excreted into breast milk and it is estimated that the baby will receive about 1% of the mother's dose; clinical significance in the newborn is unclear

**DRUG INTERACTIONS**

- Many interactions; only clinically significant ones listed below

| Class | Example | Interaction Effects |
|---|---|---|
| **Antiarrhythmics** | Quinidine, procainamide | Cardiac conduction prolonged |
| **Anticholinergic Drugs** | Antiparkinsonian agents, antihistamines, neuroleptics | Increased anticholinergic effect; may increase risk of hyperthermia |
| **Anticoagulants** | Warfarin | Increased bleeding |
| **Antidepressants (MAOIs)** | | If used together, do not add cyclic antidepressants to MAOI: start cyclic antidepressant first or simultaneously with MAOI. For patients already on MAOI, discontinue MAOI 10 to 14 days before starting combination therapy. Combined cyclic and MAOI therapy has increased antidepressant effects. Caution when fluoxetine given before or after MAOI; hypermetabolic syndrome (serotonergic) reported. |
| **Antihypertensives** | Bethanidine, clonidine, debrisoquin, guanethidine, reserpine | Decreased antihypertensive effect |
| | Acetazolamide, thiazide diuretics | Hypotension augmented |
| **CNS Depressants** | Barbiturates, hypnotics, antihistamines, alcohol, neuroleptics | Increased sedation, CNS depression |
| **Hypertensives** | Epinephrine, norepinephrine (levarterenol), phenylephrine | Enhanced pressor response |
| | Isoproterenol | May increase likelihood of arrhythmias |
| **Lithium** | | Potentiates antidepressant effect, Caution with fluoxetine; report of increased lithium level |
| **Thyroid Drugs** | Triiodothyronine ($T_3$ liothyronine), l-thyroxine ($T_4$) | Potentiates antidepressant effect |

# Monoamine Oxidase Inhibitors (MAOIs)

**INDICATIONS**

- The management of anxiety disorders in which the predominant symptom is depression
- "Atypical" depression
- Panic disorder prophylaxis
- Obsessive-compulsive neurosis
- Possible anti-herpetic effect

**PHARMACOLOGY**

- Inhibits the action of monoamine oxidase, an enzyme that metabolizes the neurohormones responsible for stimulating physical and mental activity (serotonin, epinephrine, and norepinephrine)
- Combined therapy with cyclic antidepressants or lithium may increase antidepressant effect

**DOSING**

- Best response to MAOIs occurs at dosages that reduce MAO enzyme activity by at least 80%
  May require up to 2 weeks to reach maximum MAO inhibition

**SIDE EFFECTS**

- The most common are: restlessness, insomnia, constipation, anorexia, nausea, vomiting, dry mouth, urinary retention, transient impotence, skin rash, drowsiness, headache, dizziness, weakness, orthostatic hypotension
- Occasionally, hypertensive patients may experience a rise in blood pressure

**HYPERTENSIVE CRISIS**

- Can occur due to ingestion of incompatible foods (containing elevated levels of tyramine) or drugs (see lists pp.9-10)
- Not related to dose of drug

**Signs and Symptoms**

- Occipital headache, neck stiffness or soreness, nausea, vomiting, sweating (sometimes with fever and sometimes with cold, clammy skin), dilated pupils and photophobia, sudden unexplained nose bleeds, tachycardia, bradycardia, and constricting chest pains

**Treatment**

- Withhold medication and notify physician immediately
- Phentolamine (Rogitine) can be ordered by the physician to counteract the hypertensive crisis
- Nifedipine 10 mg bitten and placed under the tongue may decrease blood pressure

**PRECAUTIONS**

- Should not be administered to patients with cerebrovascular difficulty, cardiovascular disease, or a history of hypertension
- Should not be used alone in patients with marked psychomotor agitation
- When changing from one MAOI to another, or to a tricyclic antidepressant, allow a minimum of ten medication-free days
- Need 10-14 days to be excreted from the system before an incompatible drug or food is given, or before surgery
- Hypertensive crisis can occur if given concurrently with certain drugs or foods (see lists pp. 8-9)

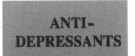

**ANTI-DEPRESSANTS**

# Monoamine Oxidase Inhibitors (MAOIs) (cont'd)

**TOXICITY**

- Symptoms same as side effects but intensified
- Severe cases progress to extreme dizziness and shock
- Overdose, whether accidental or intentional, can be fatal: patient may be symptom-free up to 6 hours, then progress to restlessness - coma - death — therefore, close medical supervision is indicated for 48 hours following an overdose

- Education of patient regarding foods and drugs to avoid is important; a diet sheet should be provided for each patient
- The incidence of orthostatic hypotension is high, especially in the elderly and at the start of treatment: tell patient to get out of bed slowly

**FOOD AND DRUG INTERACTIONS**

There are many serious food and drug interactions that may precipitate a hypertensive crisis:

Foods to avoid
- All matured or aged cheeses (Cheddar, Brick, Mozzarella, Parmesan, Blue, Gruyere, Stilton, Brie, Swiss, Camembert, etc.)
- Broad bean pods
- Meat extract (e.g., "Marmite," "Bovril," "Oxo"), concentrated yeast extracts
- Pickled herring, dried salted fish

Reactions have also been reported with
- Sour cream, yoghurt
- Soya sauce, meat tenderizers
- Caviar, snails, tinned fish
- Homemade red wine, beer, sherry
- Tea, coffee, cola
- Tinned and packet soup
- Sausage: bologna, salami, pepperoni, summer sausage, or other unrefrigerated fermented meats, game meat that has been hung
- Chocolate
- Overripe fruit, avocadoes, canned figs, raisins

It is **SAFE** to use cottage cheese, cream cheese, farmer's cheese, processed cheese, and liver (as long as they are fresh), white wine and spirits. **MAKE SURE ALL FOOD IS FRESH, STORED PROPERLY AND EATEN SOON AFTER BEING PURCHASED.** Never touch food that is fermented or possibly "off."

Over-the-counter drugs to avoid
- Cold remedies, decongestants (including nasal sprays and drops), most antihistamines and cough medicines
- Narcotic pain killers (e.g., 222s)
- All stimulants including "Pep-pills" ("Wake-ups")
- All appetite suppressants
- Anti-asthma drugs
- Sleep aids and sedatives ("Sominex")

| Class | Example | Interaction Effects |
|---|---|---|
| Anaesthetics | | May enhance CNS depression |
| Analgesics | Narcotics | Excitation, sweating, hypotension; if a narcotic is required, meperidine should not be used Other narcotics should be instituted cautiously |
| Anticholinergic agents | Antiparkinsonian agents, neuroleptics | Increased atropine-like effects |
| Anticonvulsants | Carbamazepine | Due to the structural similarity between carbamazepine and cyclic antidepressants, there is a theoretical possibility that there will be an interaction between these drugs |
| Antidepressants (cyclic) | | If used together, do not add cyclic antidepressants to MAOI. Start cyclic antidepressant first or simultaneously with MAOI. For patients already on MAOI, discontinue the MAOI for 10 to 14 days before starting combination therapy. Combined cyclic and therapy MAOI has increased antidepressant effects |
| CNS depressants | Barbiturates, sedatives, alcohol | May enhance CNS depression |
| Levodopa | | Increased blood pressure |
| L-tryptophan | | Reports of "serotonin syndrome," with hyperreflexia, tremor, myoclonic jerks, and ocular oscillations |
| Muscle relaxants | Succinylcholine | May prolong apnea |
| Sympathomimetic amines | 1. Indirect acting: amphetamine, methylphenidate, ephedrine, pseudo-ephedrine, phenylpropanolamine, dopamine, tyramine | Release of large amounts of norepinephrine with hypertensive reaction. AVOID |
| | 2. Direct acting: epinephrine, isoproterenol, norepinephrine (levarterenol), methoxamine | No interaction |
| | 3. Phenylephrine | Increased pressor response |

# Antidepressant Doses

| Drug | Therapeutic Dose Range ( mg) | Maximum Therapeutic Dose in Literature (mg) | Equivalent Dose (mg) | Suggested Plasma Level (nmol/L **) | Neurotransmitter Affected | | |
|---|---|---|---|---|---|---|---|
| **TRICYCLIC** | | | | | | | |
| Amitriptyline (Elavil) | 75 - 300 | 500 | 50 | * 400 - 800 | NE (++) | 5-HT (+++) | DA (+) |
| Clomipramine (Anafranil) | 75 - 225 | 500 | 50 | 300 - 1000 | NE (+) | 5-HT (++) | |
| Desipramine (Norpramin) | 75 - 300 | 400 | 50 | 500 - 1000 | NE (++++) | 5-HT (+++) | |
| Doxepin (Sinequan) | 75 - 300 | 350 | 50 | * 500 - 950 | NE (+) | 5-HT (++) | |
| Imipramine (Tofranil) | 75 - 300 | 750 | 50 | * 150 - 500 | NE (+++) | 5-HT (+++) | |
| Nortriptyline (Aventyl) | 40 - 200 | 400 | 25 | 150 - 500 | NE (+++) | 5-HT (+) | |
| Protriptyline (Triptil) | 30 - 60 | 150 | 15 | | NE (++++) | 5-HT (++) | |
| Trimipramine (Surmontil) | 75 - 300 | 800 | 50 | | NE (++) | 5-HT (+) | DA (+) |
| **DIBENZOXAZEPINE** | | | | | | | |
| Amoxapine (Asendin) | 100 - 400 | 900 | 100 | | NE (+++) | 5-HT (++) | DA (++) |
| **TETRACYCLIC** | | | | | | | |
| Maprotiline (Ludiomil) | 100 - 225 | 400 | 50 | 650 - 950 | NE (+++) | 5-HT (+) | |
| **TRIAZOLOPYRIDINE** | | | | | | | |
| Trazodone (Desyrel) | 150 - 40 | 600 | 100 | 2000 - 5000 | | 5-HT (++) | |
| **MONOCYCLIC** | | | | | | | |
| Bupropion (Wellbutrin)*** | 225 - 450 | 900 | | | NE (u) | | DA (u) |
| **BICYCLIC** | | | | | | | |
| Fluoxetine (Prozac) | 20 - 80 | 80 | | | | 5-HT (++++) | |
| **MAO INHIBITORS** | | | | | | | |
| Isocarboxazid (Marplan) | 30 - 50 | 80 | 10 | | NE (u) | 5-HT (u) | DA (u) |
| Phenelzine (Nardil) | 45 - 90 | 150 | 15 | | NE (u) | 5-HT (u) | DA (u) |
| Tranylcypromine (Parnate) | 20 - 60 | 300 | 10 | | NE (u) | 5-HT (u) | DA (u) |

Doses used at the Clarke Institute often fall in the range between monograph doses and maximum doses used in the literature.
Monograph doses are just a guideline, and each patient's medication must be individualized.

\*   includes sum of drug and its metabolites
\*\*  approximate conversion:  nmol/L = 3.5 x ng/mL
\*\*\* Approved but not marketed in U.S.

| | | | | | |
|---|---|---|---|---|---|
| 5-HT | = | Serotonin | High | ++++ |
| NE | = | Norepinephrine | Moderate | +++ |
| DA | = | Dopamine | Low | ++ |
| | | | Very Low | + |
| | | | Potency unknown | u |

# Frequency of Adverse Reactions of Tricyclic Antidepressants at Therapeutic Doses

| Reaction | Amitriptyline | Clomipramine | Desipramine | Doxepin | Imipramine | Nortriptyline | Protriptyline | Trimipramine |
|---|---|---|---|---|---|---|---|---|
| **ANTICHOLINERGIC EFFECTS** | | | | | | | | |
| Dry mouth | > 30% | > 30% | 10-30% | > 30% | > 30% | 10-30% | 10-30% | 10-30% |
| Blurred vision | 10-30% | 10-30% | 2-10% | 10-30% | 10-30% | 2-10% | 10-30% | 2-10% |
| Constipation | 10-30% | 10-30% | 2-10% | 10-30% | 10-30% | 10-30% | 10-30% | 10-30% |
| Sweating | 10-30% | 10-30% | 2-10% | 2-10% | 10-30% | < 2% | 10-30% | 2-10% |
| Delayed micturition * | 2-10% | 10-30% | - | < 2% | 10-30% | < 2% | < 2% | < 2% |
| **CNS EFFECTS** | | | | | | | | |
| Drowsiness, sedation | > 30% | 2-10% | 2-10% | > 30% | 10-30% | 2-10% | < 2% | > 30% |
| Insomnia | 2-10% | 10-30% | 2-10% | 2-10% | 10-30% | < 2% | 10-30% | 2-10% [b] |
| Excitement/Hypomania*** | < 2% | < 2% | 2-10% | < 2% | 10-30% | 2-10% | 10-30% | < 2% |
| Disorientation/Confusion | 10-30% | 2-10% | - | < 2% | 2-10% | 10-30% | - | 10-30% |
| Headache | 2-10% | 2-10% | < 2% | < 2% | 10-30% | < 2% | - | 2-10% |
| **EXTRAPYRAMIDAL EFFECTS** | | | | | | | | |
| Unspecified | 2-10% [a] | < 2% [a] | < 2% | 2-10% [a] | < 2% | - | - | < 2% |
| Tremor (fine) | 10-30% | 10-30% | 2-10% | 2-10% | 10-30% | 10-30% | 2-10% | 10-30% |
| **CARDIOVASCULAR EFFECTS** | | | | | | | | |
| Orthostatic hypotension/ dizziness | 10-30% | 10-30% | 2-10% | 10-30% | > 30% | 2-10% | 10-30% | 10-30% |
| Tachycardia | 10-30% | 10-30% | 10-30% | 2-10% | 10-30% | 2-10% | 2-10% | 2-10% |
| ECG changes ** | 10-30% | 10-30% | 2-10% | 2-10% | 10-30% | 2-10% | 10-30% | 10-30% |
| Cardiac arrhythmia | 2-10% | 2-10% | 2-10% | 2-10% | 2-10% | 2-10% | 2-10% | 2-10% |
| G.I. distress (nausea) | 2-10% | 2-10% | 2-10% | < 2% | 10-30% | < 2% | - | < 2% |
| Dermatitis, rash | 2-10% | 2-10% | 2-10% | < 2% | 2-10% | < 2% | < 2% | < 2% |
| Weakness, fatigue | 10-30% | 2-10% | 2-10% | 2-10% | 10-30% | 10-30% | 10-30% | 2-10% |
| Weight gain (over 6 kg) | > 30% | 10-30% | 2-10% | 2-10% | 10-30% | 2-10% | - | 10-30% |
| Sexual disturbances | 2-10% | 10-30% | 2-10% | 2-10% | 2-10% | < 2% | < 2% | - |
| Epileptic seizures [c] | < 2% | < 2% | < 2% | < 2% | < 2% | < 2% | < 2% | < 2% |

\* Primarily in the elderly   \*\* ECG abnormalities usually without cardiac injury   **(a)** Tardive dyskinesia reported (rarely)   **(b)** No effect on REM sleep   **(c)** In non-epileptic patients
\*\*\* More likely in bipolar patients   - None reported in literature perused

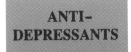

**ANTI-DEPRESSANTS**

# Frequency of Adverse Reactions of Other Classes of Antidepressants at Therapeutic Doses

| Reaction | Amoxapine | Maprotiline | Trazodone | Isocarboxazid | Phenelzine | Tranylcypromine | Bupropion [l] | Fluoxetine |
|---|---|---|---|---|---|---|---|---|
| **ANTICHOLINERGIC EFFECTS** | | | | | | | | |
| Dry mouth | > 30% | > 30% | 2-10% | 10-30% | > 30% | 10-30% | 10-30% | 10-30% |
| Blurred vision | 2-10% | 10-30% | 2-10% [m] | 2-10% | 10-30% | 2-10% | 2-10% | 10-30% |
| Constipation | > 30% | 10-30% | 2-10% | 2-10% | 10-30% | 2-10% | 2-10% | 10-30% |
| Sweating | 2-10% | 2-10% | - | < 2% | 2-10% | - | 2-10% | 10-30% |
| Delayed micturition* | 10-30% | 2-10% | < 2% | 2-10% | 2-10% | 2-10% | 2-10% | 10-30% |
| **CNS EFFECTS** | | | | | | | | |
| Drowsiness, sedation | 10-30% | 10-30% | 10-30% | 2-10% | 10-30% | 10-30% | 2-10% | 10-30% |
| Insomnia | 10-30% | < 2% | < 2% | 2-10% | 10-30% [f] | 10-30% [f] | 2-10% | 10-30% |
| Excitement/Hypomania*** | 2-10% | 2-10% | - [d] | 2-10% | 10-30% | 10-30% | 2-10% | 10-30% |
| Disorientation/Confusion | 2-10% | 2-10% | < 2% | 2-10% | 2-10% | 2-10% | 2-10% | 10-30% |
| Headache | 2-10% | < 2% | 2-10% | 10-30% | 2-10% | - | 2-10% | 10-30% |
| **EXTRAPYRAMIDAL EFFECTS** | | | | | | | | |
| Unspecified | 2-10% [a] | 2-10% | 2-10% [a] | 2-10% | 2-10% | < 2% | 2-10% | 2-10% |
| Tremor (Fine) | 2-10% | 10-30% | 2-10% | 2-10% | 10-30% | 2-10% | 2-10% | 10-30% |
| **CARDIOVASCULAR EFFECTS** | | | | | | | | |
| Orthostatic hypotension/ dizziness | 10-30% | 2-10% | 10-30% [g] | 10-30% | 10-30% | 10-30% | 2-10% | 10-30% |
| Tachycardia | 10-30% | 2-10% | 2-10% | - | 10-30% | 10-30% | < 2% | - [k] |
| ECG changes** | < 2% | < 2% | < 2% | - | - | - | < 2% | < 2% |
| Cardiac arrhythmia | < 2% | < 2% | < 2% [e] | 2-10% | - | < 2% | < 2% | < 2% |
| G.I. distress (nausea) | 2-10% | 2-10% | 10-30% | 10-30% | 10-30% | 2-10% | 2-10% | 10-30% |
| Dermatitis, rash | 10-30% | 10-30% | < 2% | 2-10% | < 2% | 2-10% | 2-10% | 2-10% |
| Weakness, fatigue | 2-10% | - | < 2% | 2-10% | < 2% | <2% | 2-10% | - |
| Weight gain (over 6 kg) | < 2% | 10-30% | 2-10% | 10-30% | 10-30% | 2-10% | < 2% [j] | - [j] |
| Sexual disturbances | 2-10% | < 2% | < 2% [h] | 2-10% | 10-30% | 2-10% | < 2% | 2-10% |
| Epileptic seizures [c] | < 2% | 2-10% [i] | < 2% | - | < 2% | - [b] | < 2% [i] | < 2% |

- not reported in literature perused
\* primarily in the elderly
** ECG abnormalities usually without cardiac injury
*** more likely in bipolar patients

(a) tardive dyskinesia reported (rarely)
(b) may have anticonvulsant activity
(c) in non-epileptic patients
(d) less likely to precipitate mania; agitation may occu
(e) patients with pre-existing cardiac disease have a 10% incidence of premature ventricular contractions
(f) especially if given in the evening

(g) less frequent if drugs given after meals
(h) priapism reported
(i) higher incidence if doses above 225 mg/day(maprotiline) and 450 mg/day (bupropion)
(j) weight loss reported
(k) decreases heart rate
(l) approved but not marketed in U.S.
(m) found to lower intraocular pressure

# NEUROLEPTICS (ANTIPSYCHOTICS)

**CLASSES**

**Phenothiazines:** Aliphatic, Piperidine, Piperazine
**Thioxanthenes**
**Butyrophenone**
**Diphenylbutylpiperidine**
**Dibenzoxazepine**
**Dihydroindolone**

**INDICATIONS**

- Treat symptoms of acute and chronic psychoses (i.e. schizophrenia, manic phase of manic-depressive psychosis, delusional disorder)

**OTHER USES**

- Anti-emetic
- An adjunct to anaesthesia, refractory hiccups
- Antipruritic, especially in neurodermatitis and pruriginous eczema
- Gilles de la Tourette syndrome (especially haloperidol and pimozide)
- Porphyria
- Possibly in the prophylaxis of cyclic mood disorders
- Agitation in depression
- Agitated dementia
- Impulsivity (pericyazine)
- Obsessive compulsive disorder (pericyazine)

**GENERAL COMMENTS**

- Significant pharmacological characteristics:
    1) Antipsychotic activity
    2) Production of extrapyramidal side effects (both reversible and tardive dyskinesia)
    3) Absence of deep coma or anaesthesia with administration of large (not toxic) doses
    4) Absence of physical or psychic dependence
- The term "tranquillizer" was introduced to describe the psychic effects of reserpine (which is rarely used for this indication now); the term is outmoded
- Neuroleptics must be distinguished from both anxiolytics and sedatives as neither of these possesses antipsychotic properties in usual doses
- Appear to control symptoms of schizophrenia such as thought disorders, hallucinations, delusions, alterations in affect, and autism

**NEUROLEPTICS**

# NEUROLEPTICS (cont'd)

**DOSES**

- See pp. 20 and 21

**PHARMACOLOGY**

- Exact mechanism of action unknown; may produce blockage of dopamine receptors in the brain — primary action is apparently a depression of the subcortical area of the brain without impairing cortical functions (dopamine blockade?)

**PHARMACOKINETICS**

- Varies with individual agents

Oral

- Peak plasma levels of oral doses reached 1-4 hours after administration
- Highly bound to plasma proteins
- Most phenothiazines and thioxanthenes have active metabolites
- Metabolized extensively in the liver
- Once-daily dosing is appropriate due to long elimination half-life

IM

- Generally peak plasma level reached sooner than with oral preparation
- Bioavailability usually higher than with oral drug; dosage should be adjusted accordingly (loxapine excepted)

Depot IM

- See chart on pp. 25-27

**ADVERSE EFFECTS**

- See chart on p. 23 for incidence of adverse effects

1. Anticholinergic Effects

- A result of antagonism at muscarinic receptors
- Common; effects are additive if given concurrently with other anticholinergic agents
- Dry mucous membranes [Management: sugar-free gum and candy, oral lubricants (e.g. MoiStir, OraCare D, etc.), pilocarpine mouth wash]
- Blurred vision, dry eyes [Management: artificial tears, wetting solutions]
- Constipation [Management: increase bulk and fluid intake, fecal softener, bulk laxative]
- Urinary retention [Management: bethanecol]

2. CNS Effects

- A result of antagonism at $H_1$-receptors
- Sedation common, especially during the first two weeks of therapy (primarily with aliphatics) [Management: prescribe bulk of dose at bedtime]
- Lowered seizure threshold; caution in patients with history of seizure
- Confusion, disturbed concentration, disorientation (more common with high doses, in elderly)
- Weight gain

### 3. Neurological Effects

- A result of antagonism at dopamine receptors
- Extrapyramidal reactions (see pp. 21 and 22) (seen primarily with the high potency neuroleptics):
  dystonias, dyskinesias, "Pisa syndrome"; akathisia; pseudoparkinsonism; perioral tremor "rabbit syndrome"
- Tardive dyskinesia (see p. 21)
  Persistent or tardive dyskinesias appear very late in therapy, rarely sooner than 3-6 months, and often persist after termination of therapy. Usually occur in the over-40 age group. Females are affected twice as often as males. Symptoms often appear only when the neuroleptic is discontinued or the dosage lowered. Symptoms are not alleviated by antiparkinsonian medication; tend to be made worse by it. Symptoms disappear during sleep and can be suppressed by intense voluntary effort and concentration; they are exacerbated by stress.
- Bucco-lingual-facial hyperkinesis: smacking and licking of lips, sucking or chewing movements, rolling and protrusion of tongue, blinking, grotesque grimaces, spastic facial distortions.
- Choreoathetoid movements of extremities: clonic jerking of fingers, ankles and toes, trunk, neck and pelvic thrusts.
- Tardive dystonia
- Tardive ballismus
- Tardive Gilles de la Tourette
- Tardive akathisia

### 4. Cardiovascular Effects

- A result of antagonism at $\alpha_1$-adrenergic and muscarinic receptors
- Hypotension, most frequent with parenteral use. **DO NOT USE EPINEPHRINE**, as it may further lower the blood pressure. Levarterenol (norepinephrine) or phenylephrine may be used
- Tachycardia, dizziness, fainting, non-specific ECG changes, in rare cases "torsade de pointes" arrhythmia have occurred (esp. with thioridazine and pimozide)

### 5. G.I. Effects

- Anorexia, dyspepsia, constipation, occasionally diarrhea
- Peculiar taste, glossitis

### 6. Endocrine Effects

- In women, moderate breast engorgement and lactation, amenorrhea, delayed ovulation, menstrual irregularities, changes in libido [Management: bromocriptine if prolactin level elevated]
- False positive pregnancy test
- In men, decreased libido, inhibition of ejaculation, gynecomastia, rarely galactorrhea [Management: bromocriptine if prolactine level elevated]
- Increased appetite, weight gain, hypoglycemia or hyperglycemia, glycosuria and high or prolonged glucose tolerance tests

### 7. Ocular Changes

- Lenticular pigmentation
  - related to long-term use of neuroleptics (primarily chlorpromazine)
  - granular deposits in eye
  - vision usually is not impaired
  - often present in patients with neuroleptic-induced skin pigmentation or photosensitivity reactions
- Pigmentary retinopathy
  - primarily associated with chronic use of thioridazine or chlorpromazine
  - reduced visual acuity (may occasionally revert if drug stopped); blindness can occur

*Continued*

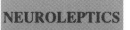

**NEUROLEPTICS**

# NEUROLEPTICS (cont'd)

*Adverse effects (cont'd )*

| **8. Hypersensitivity Reactions** |

Usually appear within the first few months of therapy (but may occur after the drug is discontinued)

- Skin reactions, rashes, abnormal skin pigmentation
- Cholestatic jaundice
    - occurs in less than 0.1% of patients within first 4 weeks of treatment; signs include yellow skin, dark urine, pruritis
    - reversible if drug stopped
- Agranulocytosis
    - occurs in less than 0.01% of patients within first 12 weeks of treatment
    - Mortality high if drug not stopped and treatment initiated
    - Signs include sore throat, fever, weakness, mouth sores
    - Rarely, asthma, laryngeal, angioneurotic or peripheral edema, and anaphylactic reactions occur
- Neuroleptic Malignant Syndrome (NMS) - rare disorder (< 1% incidence) characterized by muscular rigidity, tachycardia, hyperthermia, altered consciousness, autonomic dysfunction, and increase in CPK
    - can occur with any class of neuroleptic agent, at any dose, and at any time (more common with rapid neuroleptization, and in summer)
    - potentially fatal unless recognized early and medication is stopped.  Supportive therapy must be instituted as soon as possible

| **9. Temperature Regulations** |

- Altered ability of body to regulate response to changes in temperature and humidity; may become hyperthermic or hypothermic in temperature extremes due to inhibition of the hypothalamic control area

**PRECAUTIONS**

- Hypotension occurs most frequently with parenteral use, especially with high doses; the patient should be in supine position during I.M. administration and remain supine or seated for at least 1/2 hour.  Measure the B.P. before each I.M. dose
- I.M. injections should be very slow.  The deltoid offers faster absorption as it has better blood perfusion
- Use with caution in the elderly, in the presence of hepatic disease, cardiovascular disease, chronic respiratory disorder, hypoglycemia, convulsive disorders
- Should be used very cautiously in patients with narrow angle glaucoma or prostatic hypertrophy
- Withdrawal: abrupt cessation of high doses may rarely cause gastritis, nausea, vomiting, dizziness, tremors, feelings of warmth or cold, sweating, tachycardia, headache and insomnia in some patients. Symptoms begin 2-3 days after abrupt discontinuation of treatment and may last up to 14 days

**TOXICITY**

- Symptoms of toxicity are extensions of common adverse effects: anticholinergic, extrapyramidal, CNS stimulation followed by CNS depression
- Postural hypotension may be complicated by shock or coma, cardiovascular insufficiency, myocardial infarction and arrhythmias
- Convulsions appear late

## NURSING IMPLICATIONS

- Careful observation, data collection and documentation of patient behaviour patterns prior to drug administration, as well as during therapy, are essential nursing measures
- Nursing care is essential in minimizing side effects; patients should be educated and reassured about side effects to promote positive attitudes towards taking medication; allow patient to ventilate fears about medication
- Prn antiparkinsonian agents may be required liberally during first few weeks of treatment
- Hold dose and notify physician if patient develops severe persistent extrapyramidal reactions (longer than a few hours), or has symptoms of jaundice or blood dyscrasias (fever, sore throat, infection, cellulitis, weakness)
- Intake and output checks for urinary retention or constipation may be indicated
- Check patients on depot injections for indurations (especially with fluspirilene)
- Recommend patient visit general practitioner yearly for a physical examination, including ophthamological

## USE IN PREGNANCY

- Neuroleptics have not been clearly demonstrated to have teratogenic effects
- If possible, avoid during first trimester
- Use of moderate to high doses in last trimester may produce extrapyramidal reactions in newborn and impair temperature regulation after birth

### Breast Milk

- Neuroleptics have been detected in breast milk; clinical significance in the newborn is unclear

## ADMINISTRATION

### Short-acting Injections

- Watch for orthostatic hypotension, especially with parenteral administration; keep patient supine or seated for 1/2 hour afterwards; monitor B.P. before and after each injection
- Give I.M. into upper outer quadrant of buttocks or in the deltoid (deltoid offers faster absorption as it has better blood perfusion); alternate sites, charting (L) or (R); massage slowly after, to prevent sterile abscess formation; tell patient that injection may sting
- Prevent contact dermatitis by keeping drug solution off patient's skin and clothing
- Do not let drug stand in syringe for longer than 15 minutes as plastic may adsorb drug

### Depot Injections

- Use a dry needle (at least 21 gauge); give deep I.M. into large muscle using Z-track method; rotate sites and specify in charting
- S.C. administration can be used
- Do not let drug stand in syringe for longer than 15 minutes
- Do not massage injection site

### Oral Medication

- Protect liquids from light
- Discard markedly discoloured solutions; however, a slight yellowing does not affect potency
- Dilute with milk, orange juice or semi-solid food just before administration as some drugs may be bitter in taste
- Some liquids such as chlorpromazine and methotrimeprazine have local anaesthetic effects and should be well diluted to prevent choking
- Do not give oral medication within 2 hours of an antacid or antidiarrheal drug, as absorption of the neuroleptic will be decreased
- If patient is suspected of not swallowing tablet medication, liquid medication can be given

**NEUROLEPTICS**

# NEUROLEPTICS (cont'd)

**PATIENT INSTRUCTIONS**

- Warn patient to avoid photosensitivity reactions by using sunscreen agents and protective clothing until response to sun has been determined
- Patient should avoid exposure to extreme heat and humidity as neuroleptics affect the body's ability to regulate temperature
- Caution patient about driving a car or operating machinery until response to drug is determined. Drowsiness and dizziness usually subside after the first few weeks; patient should get up slowly from lying or sitting to avoid orthostatic hypotension. Caution should be used when combining neuroleptics with alcohol or other depressants.
- Dry mouth can be alleviated by drinking water, sucking sour candy or chewing sugarless gum. Patient should rinse mouth periodically and brush teeth regularly. Caution patient about the use of calorie-laden or caffeine-containing beverages (e.g. colas). Excess use of caffeine may cause anxiety and agitation and counteract the beneficial effects of neuroleptics.
- Blurred vision is usually transient; near vision only is affected. If severe, Pilocarpine eye drops or Neostigmine tablets may be prescribed.
- Patient should take antiparkinsonian agents (e.g. Cogentin, Kemadrin, etc.) only for the EXTRAPYRAMIDAL side effects of neuroleptics. Excess use of these agents may precipitate an anticholinergic (toxic) psychosis.
- A gain in weight may occur in some patients receiving neuroleptics either orally or by depot injection. Proper diet, exercise and avoidance of calorie-laden beverages is important.
- Monitor patient's intake and output. Urinary retention can occur, especially in the elderly. Bethanechol (Urecholine) can be used to reverse this.
- Anticholinergics reduce peristalsis and decrease intestinal secretions leading to constipation. Increasing fluids and bulk (e.g. bran, salads), as well as fruit in the diet is beneficial. If necessary, bulk laxatives (e.g. Metamucil, Prodiem) or a stool softener (e.g. Surfak) can be used.

**DRUG INTERACTIONS**

Many interactions; only clinically significant ones listed below

| Class | Example | Interaction Effects |
|---|---|---|
| Adsorbents | Antacids, activated charcoal cholestyramine, kaolin-pectin | Oral absorption decreased significantly when used simultaneously. Give at least one hour before or two hours after the neuroleptic |
| Anticholinergic agents | Antiparkinsonian drugs, antidepressants, antihistamines | Potentiate atropine-like effects causing dry mouth, blurred vision, constipation, etc. May produce inhibition of sweating, and may lead to paralytic ileus. High doses can bring on a toxic psychosis |
| CNS depressants | Antidepressants, hypnotics, antihistamines, alcohol | Will increase CNS depression |
| Epinephrine | | May result in paradoxical fall in blood pressure (due to alpha-adrenergic block produced by neuroleptics); levarterenol or phenylephrine is a safe substitute |
| Antidepressants (cyclic) | | Increased sedation, increased hypotension and increased anticholinergic effects |

# Rapid Neuroleptization

**INDICATIONS**

- Rapid control of psychotic symptomatology
- TARGET SYMPTOMS must be identified:
  - psychomotor agitation
  - physical aggression to self or others, destructiveness
  - pressure of speech, incoherency
  - delusions, hallucinations

**PROCEDURE**

- Neuroleptic injected (usually into the deltoid muscle) every 1/2 to 1 hour until symptoms controlled, e.g.:

| | | |
|---|---|---|
| Haloperidol | 5 - 10 mg | (usual drug of choice) |
| Perphenazine | 5 - 10 mg | |
| Loxapine | 25 - 50 mg | |
| Fluphenazine HCl | 2.5 - 10 mg | |
| Trifluoperazine | 1 - 5 mg | |

- Symptom control is usually achieved within 6 - 8 hours, though some patients may require up to 12 hours or more
- Drug, dose and interval must be individualized. Physician should check patient before each dose
- The end point to injections is determined by one of 4 factors:
  - 1) substantial improvement in target symptoms
  - 2) patient falls asleep
  - 3) patient experiences severe side effects, or
  - 4) patient becomes toxic

- Once target symptoms are controlled, the patient should be switched to the liquid form of the drug in a dose 1 1/2 times the injection dose given in 24 hours

**PRECAUTIONS**

- Antiparkinsonian agents should be given if required for extrapyramidal reactions. Prophylactic antiparkinsonian drug treatment may be considered in patients with a history of acute dystonic reactions
- Avoid concurrent use of other drugs as much as possible (paraldehyde — see pp. 45-46 — can occasionally be given to sedate a very agitated patient)

**NURSING IMPLICATIONS**

- B.P. and vital signs should be taken before each I.M. dose. Patient should remain supine for 1/2 hour after each injection whenever possible
- Patient should be monitored continuously for adverse effects (extrapyramidal effects, confusion, level of consciousness)
- Sites of injection (deltoid muscle) should be rotated

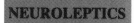

**NEUROLEPTICS**

# Neuroleptic Doses

| Drug | Equivalent Dose (mg) | Monograph Doses | Maximum Dose in Literature (mg) | Therapeutic Plasma Levels (µmol/L) [a] |
|---|---|---|---|---|
| **ALIPHATIC PHENOTHIAZINES** | | | | |
| Chlorpromazine (Largactil, Thorazine) | 100 | 30-75 mg (mild cases) [b] <br> 75-150 mg (more severe) sometimes up to 900 mg or greater | 5000 | 0.3-1.6 |
| Methotrimeprazine (Nozinan) | 70 | 6-25 mg daily for anxiety, psychosis, analgesia and sedation; for severe psychosis; doses up to 1 gm or more daily | 2200 | 0.3-1.5 |
| Triflupromazine (Vesprin) | 25 | Usual dose: I.M. 30 to 150 mg daily; oral 75 to 150 mg daily; doses over 800 mg daily have been given occasionally | 1200 | |
| **PIPERIDINE PHENOTHIAZINES** | | | | |
| Mesoridazine (Serentil) | 75 | Schizophrenia: 75-400 mg daily <br> Usual dose: 150 mg daily | 400 | |
| Pericyazine (Neuleptil) | 15 | 5-60 mg daily | 600 | |
| Pipotiazine palmitate (Piportil L4) | 0.85 (24 mg q 4 wks) | 25-250 mg q 3-4 weeks | 600/inj. | |
| Thioridazine (Mellaril) | 100 | Up to 400 mg daily; 200-800 mg daily in hospitalized patients | 2800 | 2.7-4.0 |
| **PIPERAZINE PHENOTHIAZINES** | | | | |
| Acetophenazine (Tindal) | 20 | Schizophrenia: 40-600 mg daily | | |
| Fluphenazine HC1 (Moditen, Prolixin) | 2 | Up to 20 mg daily | 1800 | 0.2-1.0 |
| Fluphenazine Enanthate (Moditen Inj., Prolixin enanthate) | 0.93 (13 mg q 2 wks) | 12.5 - 100 mg q 1-3 weeks | 1250/wk | |
| Fluphenazine Decanoate (Modecate, Prolixin decanoate) | 0.46 (13 mg q 4 wks) | 2.5 - 50 mg q 2-4 weeks | 500/wk [c] | |
| Perphenazine (Trilafon) | 10 | Outpatients: not to exceed 24 mg daily; severely disturbed hospitalized patients may temporarily require more than 24 mg daily | 256 | |
| Thioproperazine (Majeptil) | 5 | 5-40 mg daily; sometimes 90 mg or more daily is needed | | |
| Trifluoperazine (Stelazine) | 5 | Anxiety: no more than 4 mg daily [b] <br> Psychotic patients: up to 40 mg daily | 600 | 0.2-1.2 |

| | | | | |
|---|---|---|---|---|
| **THIOXANTHENES** | | | | |
| Chlorprothixene (Tarasan, Taractan) | 100 | 30-400 mg daily; greater than 600 mg daily rarely required | 2000 | |
| Flupenthixol (Fluanxol) | 5 | 3-6 mg daily as maintenance dose; up to 12 mg daily used in some patients | 320 | |
| Flupenthixol Decanoate (Fluanxol Inj.) | 1.8 (50 mg q 4 wks) | 20-80 mg q 2-3 weeks | 800/wk | |
| Thiothixene (Navane) | 3 | 15-60 mg; greater than 60 mg daily rarely increases beneficial responses | 180 | |
| **BUTYROPHENONE** | | | | |
| Haloperidol (Haldol) | 2 | 2 - 100 mg daily | 1000 | at least 40 |
| Haloperidol Decanoate (Haldol LA) | 1.1 (30 mg q 4 wks) | 50 - 400 mg q 3-4 weeks | 1200 | |
| **DIPHENYLBUTYLPIPERIDINES** | | | | |
| Fluspirilene (Imap Inj.) | 0.3 (2 mg q 1 wk) [e] (3 mg q 1 wk) [f] | 2-15 mg q 5-7 days | 60/wk | |
| Pimozide (Orap) | 2 | 2-30 mg daily | [d] 140 | |
| **DIBENZOXAZEPINE** | | | | |
| Loxapine (Loxapac, Loxitane) | 15 | 60-100 mg daily, higher than 250 mg is not recommended | 800 | |
| **DIHYDROINDOLONE** | | | | |
| Molindone (Moban) | 10 | 50-200 mg daily, usual daily dose | 400 | |

NOTE: Chlorpromazine 100 mg is used as the baseline. Equivalent doses are only approximations, i.e. they may be more applicable to acute management than to maintenance. They are more accurate in the lower dose range.
Doses used at the Clarke Institute often fall in the range between monograph doses and maximum doses used in the literature. Generally doses used are higher in the acute stage of the illness than in maintenance.
Monograph doses are just a guideline, and each patient's medication must be individualized. Plasma levels are available for neuroleptics but their clinical usefulness is limited.
The use of conversion ratios from an oral to a depot preparation is appropriate as a starting point, but wide inter-individual variations in pharmacokinetic parameters require careful clinical monitoring of the patient. It is recommended that the initially effective dose be reduced, or the injection interval increased, after 4-6 weeks to prevent possible accumulation of the drug as plasma concentrations approach steady-state.

(a) approximate conversion: $\mu$mol/L = 3 x mg/L; nmol/L = 3 x ng/ml   (c) Doses used at the Clarke Institute of Psychiatry   (e) for females. Source: *Journal of Clinical Psychopharmacology, 6(1)*, 1986
(b) neuroleptics are usually not recommended for treatment of anxiety   (d) monitor cardiac function in doses above 20 mg/day   (f) for males. Source: *Journal of Clinical Psychopharmacology, 6(1)*, 1986

**NEUROLEPTICS**

# Neurological Effects

|  | Extrapyramidal Effects | Tardive Dyskinesia |
|---|---|---|
| **Onset** | Acute or insidious (within 1 - 30 days) | After months or years of treatment, especially if drug dose decreased or discontinued |
| **Proposed Mechanism** | Due to decreased dopamine | Supersensitivity of postsynaptic dopamine receptors induced by long-term neuroleptic blockade |
| **Treatment** | Respond to antiparkinsonian drugs | Antiparkinsonian drugs generally worsen tardive dyskinesia<br>Other treatments unsatisfactory; some are aimed at balancing dopaminergic and cholinergic systems. Can mask symptoms by further suppressing dopamine with neuroleptics. Pimozide or loxapine may least aggravate tardive dyskinesia. |

# Extrapyramidal Effects

| Type | Onset | Risk Group | Clinical Course | Treatment |
|---|---|---|---|---|
| **1) Dystonias**<br>(Torsions, twisting and drawing of muscle groups; muscle spasms)<br>e.g. oculogyric crisis, laryngospasm, torticollis | Acute (usually within first 5 days) | Young male | Acute, painful, spasmodic<br>Oculogyria may be recurrent | I.M. benztropine, I.M. diphenhydramine, sublingual lorazepam<br>If symptoms recur, oral antiparkinsonian agents can be used |
| **2) Akathisia**<br>(Motor restlessness) | Insidious to acute (within 10 days) | 12-45% of patients on neuroleptics; elderly female has highest risk | May continue through entire treatment | Oral antiparkinsonian drug<br>Oral diazepam, propranolol, nadolol, pindolol<br>Reduce or change neuroleptic |
| **3) Pseudoparkinsonism**<br>(Stiffness, shuffling, mask-like facies, tremor, akinesia, rigidity) | Insidious to acute (within 30 days) | 12-45% of patients on neuroleptics; elderly female has highest risk | May continue through entire treatment | Oral antiparkinsonian drug<br>Reduce or change neuroleptic |

# Neurological Side Effects

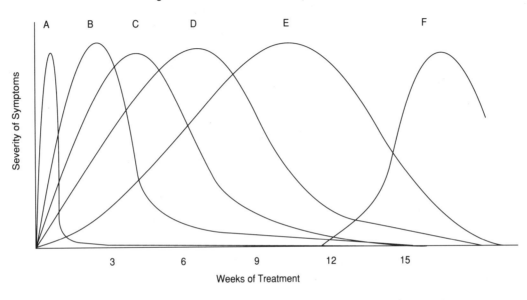

Neurological Side Effects of Neuroleptics

A : Dystonic reactions:  uncoordinated spastic movements of muscle groups (e.g. trunk, tongue, face)

B : Akinesia:  decreased muscular movements

C : Rigidity:  coarse muscular movement; loss of facial expression

D : Tremors:  fine movement (shaking) of the extremities

E : Akathisia:  restlessness, pacing (may result in insomnia)

F : Tardive Dyskinesia:  buccolinguo-masticatory syndrome, choreoathetoid  movements

(Reference:  Adapted from  DiMascio, A. & Sovner, R.D. (1976). Neuroleptic extrapyramidal side effects. *Drug Therapy*, *Oct.*, 99-103.)

**NEUROLEPTICS**

# Frequency of Adverse Reactions of Oral Neuroleptics

| Reaction | Phenothiazines | | | Thioxan-thenes | Butyro-phenone | Diphenylbutyl-piperidine | Dibenzox-azepine | Dihydro-indolone |
|---|---|---|---|---|---|---|---|---|
| | Aliphatic | Piperazine | Piperidine | | | | | |
| Drowsiness, sedation | > 30% | 2-10% | 10-30% | 10-30% | 2-10% | 10-30% | > 30% | > 30% |
| **EXTRAPYRAMIDAL EFFECTS** | | | | | | | | |
| Parkinsonism | 10-30% | > 30% | 2-10% | > 30% (b) | > 30% | 10-30% | > 30% | > 30% |
| Akathisia | 2-10% | > 30% | 2-10% | > 30% (b) | > 30% | 10-30% | > 30% | > 30% |
| Dystonic reactions | 2-10% | 10-30% | < 2% | 10-30% | > 30% | 10-30% | 10-30% | > 30% |
| **CARDIOVASCULAR EFFECTS** | | | | | | | | |
| Orthostatic hypotension | > 30% | 2-10% | 10-30% | > 30% | 2-10% | 10-30% | 10-30% | 2-10% |
| Tachycardia | 10-30% | 2-10% | 2-10% | 2-10% | < 2% | 2-10% | 10-30% | < 2% |
| ECG abnormalities ** | 10-30% | 2-10% | 10-30% (d) | 2-10% | < 2% | 2-10% (e) | < 2% | < 2% |
| Cardiac arrhythmias | 2-10% | - | 10-30% (d) | < 2% | < 2% | < 2% (e) | - | - |
| **ANTICHOLINERGIC EFFECTS** | 10-30% | 2-10% | 10-30% | 10-30% | 10-30% | 10-30% | 10-30% | 10-30% |
| **ENDOCRINE EFFECTS** | | | | | | | | |
| Inhibition of ejaculation | 2-10% | 2-10% | 10-30% | < 2% | < 2% | - | 2-10% | - |
| Weight gain | > 30% | 2-10% | 10-30% | 10-30% | < 2% | 2-10% | < 2% (c) | < 2% (c) |
| **SKIN REACTIONS** | | | | | | | | |
| Photosensitivity | 2-10% | 2-10% | 2-10% | < 2% | < 2% | < 2% | < 2% | - |
| Rashes | 2-10% | < 2% | 10-30% | 10-30% | < 2% | 2-10% | 2-10% | 2-10% |
| Abnormal skin pigmentation (a) | 10-30% | < 2% | 2-10% | < 2% | < 2% | - | - | - |
| **OCULAR EFFECTS** (a) | | | | | | | | |
| Lenticular pigmentation | 2-10% | < 2% | 2-10% | 2-10% | < 2% | < 2% | < 2% | - |
| Pigmentary retinopathy | 2-10% | < 2% | 10-30% | - | - | - | - | - |
| Blood dyscrasias | 2-10% | < 2% | 2-10% | < 2% | < 2% | - | < 2% | < 2% |
| Cholestatic jaundice | < 2% | < 2% | < 2% | < 2% | < 2% | - | < 2% | < 2% |
| Cholestatic jaundice | < 2% | < 2% | < 2% | < 2% | < 2% | < 2% | < 2% | - |
| Epileptic seizures | 2-10% | < 2% | < 2% | 2-10% | < 2% | 2-10% | < 2% | < 2% |

- none reported in literature perused
** ECG abnormalities usually without cardiac injury

(a) usually seen after prolonged use
(b) mainly with thiothixene

(c) weight loss reported
(d) thioridazine above 800 mg daily poses greater risk

(e) pimozide above 20 mg daily poses greater risk

# A Comparison of Depot Neuroleptics

| | Flupenthixol Decan. (Fluanxol) | Fluphenazine Enanthate (Moditen; Prolixin) | Fluphenazine Decanoate (Modecate; Prolixin) | Fluspirilene (Imap) | HaloperidolDecanoate (Haldol LA) | Pipotiazine Palmitate (Piportil L4) |
|---|---|---|---|---|---|---|
| **Chemical Class** | Thioxanthene | Piperazine pheno-thiazine | Piperazine pheno-thiazine | Diphenylbutyl-piperidine | Butyrophenone | Piperidine pheno-thiazine |
| **Form** | Esterified with a 10-carbon chain fatty acid and dissolved in vegetable oil. Must be hydrolyzed to free flupenthixol. Metabolites inactive. | Esterified with a 7-carbon chain fatty acid and dissolved in sesame oil. Must be hydrolyzed to free fluphenazine. | Esterified with a 10-carbon chain fatty acid and dissolved in sesame oil. Must be hydrolyzed to free fluphenazine. | Drug in a microcrystal-line form in an aqueous suspension. Immediately active on injection.Does not have to be hydro-lyzed. | Esterified with a 10-carbon chain fatty acid and dissolved in sesame oil. Must be hydrolyzed to free haloperidol. | Esterified with palmitic acid in sesame oil. Must be hydrolyzed to free to pipothiazine. |
| **Strength supplied** | 2% - 20 mg/ml 10% - 100 mg/ml | 25 mg/ml | 25 mg/ml 100 mg/ml (investigational) | 2 mg/ml 10 mg/ml | 50 mg/ml 100 mg/ml | 25 mg/ml 50 mg/ml |
| **Usual dose range** | 20 - 80 mg | 25 - 100 mg | 12.5 - 50 mg | 2 - 10 mg | 50 - 300 mg | 50 - 300 mg |
| **Maximum dose in literature** | 800 mg/week | 1250 mg/wk (Dencker) | 400 mg/week (Clarke) | 60 mg/week (Clarke) | 1200 mg/injection (Chouinard) | 600 mg/injection |
| **Usual duration of action** | 3 weeks | 2 weeks | 4 weeks | 1.5 weeks | 4 weeks | 4 weeks |
| **Dose equivalency to 100 mg CPZ (approximate)** | 1.8 mg (50 mg q 4 wks) | 0.93 mg/day (13 mg q 2 weeks) | 0.46 mg/day (13 mg q 4 weeks) | 0.3 mg/day (2 mg q 1 wk, females, 3 mg q 1 wk, males) | (1.1 mg/day) (30 mg q 4 wks) | 0.85 mg/day (24 mg q 4 weeks) |
| **PHARMACOKINETICS** **Onset of action** | 24 - 72 hours | 24 - 96 hrs | Approx. 4 hrs | Within a few days | 48 - 72 hrs | |
| **Peak plasma level** | 4 - 7 days | 2 - 5 days | Within a few hrs | Within 24 hrs | 3 - 9 days | Approx. 4 days |
| **Elimination half-life** | 8 days (after single injection) 17 days (multiple dosing) | 3 1/2 - 4 days (after single injection) | 6 - 10 days (single injection) 14.3 days (multiple dosing) | Approx. 9 days. Slowly excreted: less than 50% in 7 days, (approx. 70 % of drug excreted in 27 days) | 18 - 21 days | 6 - 11 days (rat), 8-9 days (dog). Approx. 10% of peak plasma drug level still detectable in plasma 45 days after an injection |

**NEUROLEPTICS**

# A Comparison of Depot Neuroleptics  (cont'd)

| Adverse Effects | Flupenthixol Decan. (Fluanxol) | Fluphenazine Enanthate (Moditen; Prolixin) | Fluphenazine Decanoate (Modecate; Prolixin) | Fluspirilene (Imap) | Haloperidol Decanoate (Haldol LA) | Pipotiazine Palmitate (Piportil L4) |
|---|---|---|---|---|---|---|
| CNS | Alerting effect can cause excitation | Both drowsiness and insomnia reported | Both drowsiness and insomnia reported | Low sedative potential. Insomnia has been reported. | Both drowsiness and insomnia reported | Low sedative potential Excitation reported in approximately 12% of patients. |
| Extrapyramidal | Frequent | More frequent than with decanoate (30 - 50% of patients) | Frequent | Occasional | Frequent, however, reported less often than with oral haloperidol | Frequent, especially if dose over 100 mg q 4 weeks |
| Cardiovascular | Hypotension not reported | Hypotension and occasionally hypertension reported (usually at start of therapy) | Hypotension occurs occasionally | Hypotension and occasionally hypertension reported | Occasional hypotension: severe orthostatic hypotension not reported | Occasional hypotension |
| Anticholinergic symptoms | Uncommon | More anticholinergic than fluphenazine decanoate | Occasional | Occasional | Occasional | Frequent |
| Skin and local reactions | Indurations rarely seen (at high doses). Photosensitivity and hyperpigmentation very rare. Dermatological reactions seen | No indurations reported. Dermatological reactions have been reported | 1 case of induration seen at a high dose. Dermatological reactions have been reported | Indurations commonly reported at high doses or prolonged use. Dermatological changes reported | Inflammation at injection site. 1 case of photosensitization reported; "tracking" reported | No indurations reported. Dermatological changes reported |
| Eye changes | None reported | None reported | 11 of 63 patients on 5 years treatment showed lens and/or corneal opacities (10 were previously treated with CPZ and/or thioridazine) | None reported | None reported | None reported |

| | | | | | | |
|---|---|---|---|---|---|---|
| **Endocrine effects** | Galactorrhea, elevation in serum prolactin, impotence, loss of libido & sexual excitement | Disturbances in menstruation, amenorrhea and galactorrhea reported | Disturbances in menstruation, amenorrhea and galactorrhea reported | | Disturbances in menstruation, amenorrhea and galactorrhea reported | Menstrual irregularities, galactorrhea, amenorrhea, impotence and changes in libido reported |
| **Weight changes** | Weight gain common in 10% of patients, body weight increased by 10% | Weight gain frequently reported | Weight gain reported; 11% of patients had increased body weight by 10% | Weight gain reported | Both weight loss and weight gain reported | Weight changes reported; one study showed no increase in body weight over 3 years |
| **Laboratory changes** | Within normal variation | No hepatotoxicity. Haematological changes within normal variation. Some ECG changes seen. | One case of jaundice reported. Haematological changes within normal variation. ECG changes seen in some patients | Increases in alk. phosph., SGOT, LDH and BUN have been seen. Haematological changes within normal variation. ECG changes seen in some patients | Within normal variation | Transient changes in liver function studies seen. Haemolytic, renal and ECG within normal variation. |
| **Effect on Mood** | Mood elevating effect in low doses | May increase the risk of depression in vulnerable patients | May increase the risk of depression in vulnerable patients | | | May increase the risk of depression in vulnerable patients (not frequently reported) |
| **Use in pregnancy** | No evidence of teratogenicity in animals or humans | Single report of infant born with multiple anomalies (first trimester exposure also to doxylamine) | No evidence of teratogenicity; extrapyramidal disorder seen in infants after delivery | No teratogenic or embryotoxic effects in animals | No evidence of teratogenicity | No teratogenicity and low toxicity seen in animals |

**NEUROLEPTICS**

# ANTIPARKINSONIAN AGENTS

**INDICATIONS**

To relieve the neurological (muscular) side effects induced by neuroleptics (see pp. 30-31 for comparison of drugs):

- dyskinesias, dystonias
- pseudoparkinsonian effects (tremor, rigidity, shuffling)
- akathisia
- akinesia (muscle weakness)
- "rabbit syndrome", "Pisa syndrome"

**ADVERSE EFFECTS**

(Related to anticholinergic action)

- Common : dry mouth, blurred vision, constipation, urinary retention, skin flushing
- CNS effects:  seen primarily in the elderly and at high doses.  Includes stimulation,  disorientation, confusion, hallucinations, restlessness, weakness, incoherence
- Cardiovascular:  palpitations, tachycardia
- G.I.: nausea, vomiting

**PRECAUTIONS**

- Use cautiously in patients in whom excess anticholinergic activity could be harmful, e.g. prostatic hypertrophy, urinary retention, narrow-angle glaucoma
- Use with caution in patients with respiratory difficulties, as antiparkinsonians can dry bronchial secretions and make breathing more difficult

**NURSING IMPLICATIONS**

- Antiparkinsonian drugs should be given only to relieve extrapyramidal side effects of neuroleptics
- Some side effects of these drugs (i.e. anticholinergic) are additive to those of neuroleptics; observe patient for signs of side effects or toxicity
- Excess use/abuse of these drugs may lead to an anticholinergic (toxic) psychosis with  symptoms of disorientation, confusion, euphoria, stereotypic behaviour, in addition to physical signs such as dry mouth, blurred vision, dry flushed skin
- Monitor patient's intake and output.  Urinary retention can occur, especially in the elderly.  Bethanechol (Urecholine) can be used to reverse this problem
- To help prevent gastric irritation, administer drug after meals
- Relieve dry mouth by giving patient cool drinks, ice chips, sugarless chewing gum or hard  sour candy.  Suggest frequent rinsing of the mouth, and teeth should be brushed regularly. Patients should avoid calorie-laden beverages and sweet candy as they not  only increase the likelihood of dental caries, but will also promote weight gain.  Formerly well-fitting dentures may become ill-fitting, and can cause rubbing and/or ulceration of the gums. Products that promote or replace salivation (e.g. MoiStir, Saliment) may be of benefit
- Blurring of near vision is due to paresis of the ciliary muscle.  This can be helped by wearing suitable glasses, reading by a bright light or, if severe, by the use of Pilocarpine eye drops
- Dry eyes may be of particular difficulty to the elderly or those wearing contact lenses. Artificial tears or wetting solutions may be of benefit in dealing with this problem
- Anticholinergics reduce peristalsis and decrease intestinal secretions, leading to constipation.  Increasing fluids and bulk (e.g. bran, salads) as well as fruit in the diet is beneficial.  If necessary, bulk laxatives (e.g. Metamucil, Prodiem) or a stool softener (e.g. Surfak) can be used
- Warn the patient not to drive a car or operate machinery until response to the drug has been determined
- Appropriate patient education regarding medication and side effects is necessary prior to discharge
- If akathisia does not respond to standard antiparkinsonian agents, diphenhydramine, propranolol, lorazepam or diazepam can be tried

# Effects of Drugs on Extrapyramidal Symptoms *

| Antiparkinsonian Agent | Tremor | Rigidity | Dystonia (Oculogyria) | Akinesia | Akathisia |
|---|---|---|---|---|---|
| Amantadine (Symmetrel) | ++ | +++ | ++ | +++ | ++ |
| Benztropine (Cogentin) | ++ | +++ | +++ | ++ | ++ |
| Biperiden (Akineton) | | ++ | | ++ | |
| B-blockers (propranolol, nadolol) | | | | | +++ |
| Diazepam (Valium) | | ++ | +++ | | +++ |
| Diphenhydramine (Benadryl) | ++ | + | ++ | | +++ |
| Ethopropazine (Parsitan) | +++ | ++ | + | | ++ |
| Lorazepam (Ativan) | | + | +++ | | ++ |
| Orphenadrine (Disipal) | ++ | + | | | |
| Procyclidine (Kemadrin) | + | ++ | ++ | ++ | + |
| Trihexyphenidyl (Artane) | + | ++ | ++ | ++ | |

\* based on literature and clinical observations
- no effect     + some effect (20% response)          ++ moderate effect (20-40% response)          +++ good effect (> 40% response)

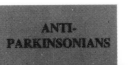

**ANTI-PARKINSONIANS**

# Comparison of Antiparkinsonian Agents

| Antiparkinsonian Agents | Equivalent Dose (mg) | Therapeutic Effects | Adverse Effects | Dose |
|---|---|---|---|---|
| Amantadine (Symmetrel) | 50 | May improve akathisia, akinesia, rigidity, dystonia, parkinsonism, and tardive dyskinesia<br>May enhance the effects of other antiparkinsonian agents<br>Tolerance to fixed dose may develop after 1-8 weeks<br>Less anticholinergic than other agents | Common: indigestion, nervous excitement, difficulty in concentration, dizziness<br>Less often: skin rash, tremors, slurred speech, ataxia, psychic depression, insomnia and lethargy (these are dose-related and disappear on drug withdrawal) | Orally: 100 to 400 mg daily |
| **Antihistamines**<br>**Diphenhydramine** (Benadryl) | 25 | Has effect on tremor<br>Added sedative effect, which may benefit tension and excitation<br>May enhance the effects of other antiparkinsonian agents | Somnolence and confusion, especially in the elderly | IM/IV: 25-50 mg for dystonia<br>Orally: 25-50 mg q.i.d. |
| Orphenadrine (Disipal) | 25 | Some effect on rigidity<br>Mild stimulant<br>Modest effect on sialorrhea<br>Beneficial effects tend to wear off in 2-6 months | Slight dryness of mouth, sedation, mild central excitation | Orally: 50 mg t.i.d. up to 400 mg/day |
| **Benzodiazepines**<br>**Diazepam** (Valium, etc.) | 5 | Beneficial effect on akathisia and dystonia<br>Muscle relaxant | Drowsiness, lethargy | IV: 10 mg for dystonia by slow direct IV push (rate of 5 mg (1mL)/min)<br>Orally: 2-5 mg t.i.d. |
| Lorazepam (Ativan) | 1 | Beneficial effect on akathisia and dystonia | As above | Sublingual: 1-2 mg up to t.i.d.<br>IM: 1-2 mg for dystonia |

| | | | | |
|---|---|---|---|---|
| **Benztropine**<br>(Cogentin) | 0.5 | Beneficial effect on rigidity<br>Relieves sialorrhea and drooling<br>Powerful muscle relaxant and sedative<br>Cumulative and long-acting; once-daily dosing can be used<br>No cerebral stimulating action<br>IM/IV: dramatic effect on dystonic symptoms | Dry mouth, blurred vision, urinary retention,<br>   constipation<br>Increases intraocular pressure<br>Toxic psychosis when abused or overused | Orally: 1-2 mg b.i.d.<br>  up to 6 mg b.i.d if<br>  needed.<br>  IM/IV: 1-2 mg.<br>May repeat in 30<br>minutes. |
| **Biperiden**<br>(Akineton) | 0.5 | Has effect against rigidity and akinesia | As for benztropine<br>May cause euphoria and increased tremor | Orally: 2-6 mg up<br>  to t.i.d. |
| **Ethopropazine**<br>(Parsitan) | 50 | Has effect against rigidity; improves posture, gait<br>  and speech<br>Specific for tremor | Dry mouth, postural dizziness, somnolence and<br>  confusion can occur<br>Safe to use in moderate doses in patients with glaucoma | Initial oral dose: 50 mg<br>  t.i.d. up to 400 mg<br>  per day. In major<br>tremor start with<br>100 mg t.i.d. and may<br>increase to 600-900<br>mg/day. |
| **Piperidine Agents**<br>Procyclidine<br>(Kemadrin) | 1.5 | Similar to trihexyphenidyl<br>Milder and questionable effect on tremor<br>Useful agent to use in combination when muscle<br>  rigidity is severe<br>Strong cerebral stimulating action | Less pronounced side effects than with trihexyphenidyl<br>Slight blurring of vision, giddiness in some patients | Starting oral dose:<br>2.5 mg b.i.d<br>Usual daily dose:<br>5 - 60 mg |
| Trihexyphenidyl<br>(Artane) | 1 | Mild to moderate effect against rigidity and spasm<br>  (occasionally get dramatic results)<br>Tremor alleviated to a lesser degree; as a result of relaxing<br>  muscle spasm, more tremor activity may be noted.<br>Cerebral stimulating action — can be used during the<br>  day for sluggish, lethargic and akinetic patients | Dry mouth, blurred vision, G.I. distress<br>Less sedating potential<br>Severe and persistent mental confusion may occur,<br>  especially in the elderly; must recognize this as a<br>  toxic state<br>At toxic doses get restless, delirium, hallucinations; these<br>  disappear when the drug is discontinued (most anti-<br>  cholinergic of the antiparkinsonian agents — liable to<br>  be abused) | Orally: 4 - 15 mg<br>  daily, up to 30 mg<br>tolerated in younger<br>patients |

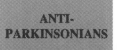

**ANTI-PARKINSONIANS**

# ANXIOLYTICS

**CLASSES**

(according to chemical similarities)

### Barbiturates and Carbamates

Both act as CNS depressants; seldom used as anxiolytics because:

a) they are habit-forming, causing physical dependence
b) they can have severe withdrawal symptoms
c) tolerance develops quickly, requiring increased dosage
d) they have a low margin of safety (therapeutic dose close to toxic dose)
e) the barbiturates have many drug interactions

### Antihistamine Sedatives

e.g. Hydroxyzine (Atarax)

A CNS depressant with few side effects; used primarily for itching of psychogenic origin

### Benzodiazepines

Most commonly used anxiolytic agents

### Azaspirodecanedione

e.g. Buspirone (Buspar)

**INDICATIONS**

- Psychoneurotic states characterized by anxiety, tension and agitation
- Management of acute and chronic alcohol withdrawal syndromes
- Convulsions: status epilepticus, petit mal, infantile spasms
- Insomnia and certain sleep disorders
- Muscle spasms, dystonia, "restless legs" syndrome
- Akathisia due to neuroleptic agents
- I.V.: sedation in severe agitation
- In mania used concomitantly with neuroleptic or lithium to control manic agitation
- Other: cardioversion, endoscopy and bronchoscopy, enhancement of analgesia during labour and delivery, pre-operative sedation
- Panic and phobic disorders (alprazolam, clonazepam)

**PHARMACOLOGY**

- Depress the CNS at the levels of the limbic system, the brain stem reticular formation and the cortex
- Benzodiazepines bind to the benzodiazepine-GABA-chloride receptor complex, facilitating the action of GABA (an inhibitory neuro-transmitter) on CNS excitability

## COMPARISON OF THE BENZODIAZEPINES

**1) Short-acting**

a) Alprazolam (Xanax)
b) Bromazepam (Lectopam)
c) Halazepam (Paxipam)
d) Lorazepam (Ativan)
e) Oxazepam (Serax)
f) Temazepam (Restoril)
g) Triazolam (Halcion)

**2) Long-acting**

a) Chlordiazepoxide (Librium)
b) Clonazepam (Rivotril)
c) Clorazepate (Tranxene)
d) Diazepam (Valium)
e) Flurazepam (Dalmane)
f) Ketazolam (Loftran)
g) Nitrazepam (Mogadon)
h) Prazepam (Centrax)

## PHARMACOKINETICS

- Well absorbed from GI tract after oral administration
- Marked inter-individual variation (up to tenfold) is found in all pharmacokinetic parameters. Age, smoking, liver disease, physical disorders as well as concurrent use of other drugs may influence parameters by changing the volume of distribution and elimination half-life of these drugs.
- There is no significant correlation between plasma concentration and clinical effects (or side effects), so plasma level monitoring is of no clinical benefit.
- Differences in pharmacokinetics between the various benzodiazepines has been presumed to indicate clinical differences as well: this is not necessarily so. However, present rationale for selection of a benzodiazepine remains the difference in pharmacokinetic profile. Generally, short-acting agents can be used as hypnotics and for acute problems relating to anxiety, while long-acting agents can be used for chronic conditions where a continuous drug effect is needed.
- It is suggested that the longer the half-life of a benzodiazepine, the greater the likelihood that the compound will have an adverse effect on daytime functioning (e.g. hangover). However, with shorter half-life benzodiazepines, withdrawal and anxiety between doses (rebound) and anterograde amnesia are seen more often.

ANXIOLYTICS

# ANXIOLYTICS (cont'd)

**ADVERSE EFFECTS**

- Are few, and often disappear with adjustment of dosage
- CNS depression — most common are extensions of the generalized sedative effect, e.g. fatigue, drowsiness, nystagmus, dysarthria, muscle weakness
- Anticholinergic effects, e.g. blurred vision (mild)
- Paradoxical agitation — insomnia, hallucinations, nightmares, rage reactions, violent behaviour; most likely in patients with a history of aggressive behaviour or unstable emotional behaviour (not seen with oxazepam)
- Confusion and disorientation — primarily in the elderly. Periods of blackouts or amnesia have been reported
- Few documented allergies to benzodiazepines

**WITHDRAWAL**

- To withdraw a patient from a benzodiazepine, an equivalent dose of diazepam should be substituted and withdrawal done according to the following protocol:

**Protocol**

1) Reduce diazepam by 10 mg daily until a total daily dose of 20 mg is reached
2) Then reduce by 5 mg daily to an end point of total abstinence (see reference 3 for this chapter). Propranolol may aid in withdrawal process

☞ This protocol is ineffective for alprazolam, which must be decreased by 0.5 mg weekly
The diazepam substitution method should not be used. Carbamazepine (in therapeutic doses) may aid in withdrawal process

**PRECAUTIONS**

- Administer with caution to elderly or debilitated patients, those with liver disease (oxazepam and lorazepam excepted), and to patients performing hazardous tasks requiring mental alertness or physical coordination

**TOXICITY**

- Rarely if ever fatal when taken alone; may be lethal when taken in combination with other drugs, such as alcohol and barbiturates
- Symptoms of overdose include hypotension, depressed respiration and coma

**NURSING IMPLICATIONS**

- Sedation is an expected effect, therefore the nurse must assess the anxiety level of patients on these drugs to determine if anxiety control has been accomplished or if over-sedation has occurred
- Inform patients that activities requiring mental alertness should be avoided
- Caution patients not to use other CNS depressant drugs (e.g. antihistamines or alcohol) without consulting the doctor
- Excessive consumption of caffeinated beverages will counteract the effects of anxiolytics
- Tolerance and physical addiction can occur and withdrawal symptoms can be produced with abrupt discontinuation after prolonged use

## USE IN PREGNANCY

- Some studies suggest an association between benzodiazepine use and teratogenicity; data are not conclusive
- High dose use by mother in third trimester may precipitate withdrawal reaction in newborn

### Breast Milk

- Benzodiazepines are excreted into breast milk in levels sufficient to produce effects in the newborn

## HAZARDS OF USE

- Anxiolytics lower the tolerance to alcohol, and high doses may produce mental confusion similar to alcohol intoxication
- Can cause physical and psychological dependence, tolerance, and withdrawal symptoms correlated to dose and duration of use
- Withdrawal symptoms resemble those of alcohol and barbiturates, e.g. tremor, agitation, headache, nausea, delirium, hallucinations, metallic taste. Abrupt withdrawal following prolonged use of high doses can produce grand-mal seizures (especially with alprazolam)

## ADMINISTRATION

- Following I.V. administration of diazepam or chlordiazepoxide, local pain and thrombophlebitis may occur due to precipitation of the drug, or due to an irritant effect of propylene glycol; I.V. diazepam emulsion (Diazemuls), is less likely to cause this problem
- I.M. use is discouraged with chlordiazepoxide and diazepam as absorption is slow, erratic and possibly incomplete; local pain often occurs. Lorazepam I.M. is adequately absorbed.

**ANXIOLYTICS**

# A Comparison of the Benzodiazepines

| Drug | Equivalent Dose (mg) ** | Peak Plasma Level p.o. | Elimination Half-life | Metabolites (m = main metabolite) | Comments | Clinically Significant Interactions | Clinical Considerations |
|---|---|---|---|---|---|---|---|
| Alprazolam | 0.5 | 1 - 2 hrs | 9 - 20 hrs | 29 metabolites; principal ones are:<br>α-hydroxyalprazolam<br>desmethylalprazolam<br>4-hydroxyalprazolam | Rapidly and completely absorbed<br>80% protein bound<br>α-hydroxyalprazolam is active | Probably similar to diazepam | Use: anxiolytic<br>    sedative<br>    alcohol withdrawal<br>    depression charac-<br>      terized by anxiety<br>Panic attack prophylaxis<br>t.i.d. dosing recommended<br>Increases stage 2, and<br>    decreases stages 1 & 4<br>    and REM sleep<br>Caution on withdrawal |
| Bromazepam | 3.0 | 0.5 - 4 hrs | 12 hrs mean | 3-hydroxybromazepam (8 - 19 hrs) | Metabolite reported to have anxiolytic activity | CNS depressants: increased effect on the CNS * | Use: anxiolytic<br>    Not recommended for use<br>    in patients with depressive<br>    disorders or psychoses * |
| Chlordiaz-epoxide | 25.0 | 1 - 4 hrs | 14 hrs mean (4 - 29 hrs parent drug) (28 - 100 hrs metabolites) | desmethylchlor-diazepoxide (m)<br>demoxepam<br>desoxydemoxepam | Volume of distribution (Vd) significantly larger in young females than males<br>Elimination half-life pro-longed and total plasma clearance decreased in elderly men (less so in elderly women) | Antacids:* decrease absorption in GI tract, but do not influence com-pleteness of absorption<br>Cimetidine:* increases blood levels of chlordia-zepoxide by decreasing elimination | Use: anxiolytic<br>    sedative<br>    alcoholism treatment<br>2 to 3-fold increase in<br>    half-life seen in patients<br>    with cirrhosis |
| Clonazepam | 0.25 | 1 - 4 hrs | 34 hrs mean (19 - 60 hrs) | No active metabolite | Quickly and completely absorbed | | Use: anticonvulsant, mostly<br>    in childhood seizures such<br>    as myoclonic infantile<br>    spasms and absences<br>Panic attack prophylaxis<br>Manic episode of B.A.D. |
| Clorazepate dipotassium | 10.0 | variable | 1.3 - 96 hrs metabolites | N-desmethyldiazepam (m) | Hydrolyzed in the stomach to active metabolite (parent compound inactive)<br>Rate of hydrolysis depends on gastric acidity, therefore absorption is unreliable (one study disputes this) | Antacids & Sodium Bicar-bonate: reduce the rate and extent of appearance of active metabolite in the blood | Use: anxiolytic |

| Drug | Dose** | Peak plasma | Half-life | Metabolites | Comments | Interactions | Use/Sleep effects |
|---|---|---|---|---|---|---|---|
| Diazepam | 5 | 1 - 2 hrs | 32 hrs mean 14 - 61 hrs (parent drug) 50 - 150 hrs (metabolites) | N-desmethyldiazepam (m) | In males has shorter half-life and higher clearance rate than in females<br>Elimination half-life prolonged and plasma clearance decreased in elderly males (less so in females)<br>Less protein-bound in elderly, therefore attain higher serum levels<br>Lipophilic; has a rapid onset of action<br>Steady state can be maintained with once-daily dosing | Smoking: associated with higher diazepam clearance especially in young<br>Food: reduces rate of drug absorption, but produces a slight increase in the extent of absorption<br>Cimetidine: increases blood levels of diazepam by 38%<br>Digoxin: diazepam increases binding of digoxin by 15%, moderately increases its half-life in plasma, and substantially decreases its excretion | Use: anxiolytic<br>sedative<br>anticonvulsant (Status epilepticus)<br>alcoholism treatment<br>akathisia<br>muscle relaxant<br>2 to 3-fold increase in half-life seen in patients with cirrhosis<br>Increases stage 2, and decreases stages 1 & 4 and REM sleep |
| Flurazepam | 15 | | 65 hrs mean (47 - 100) | N-desalkylflurazepam (m) | Rapidly metabolized to active metabolite<br>Elderly males accumulate metabolite more than young males | | Use: anxiolytic<br>sedative<br>Decreases stage 1 and increases stage 2 of sleep; no effect on REM<br>Increase in daytime sedation over time |
| Halazepam | 40 | 1 - 3 hrs | 14 hrs mean (parent) 30 - 60 hrs (metabolites) | N-desmethyldiazepam 3-hydroxyhalazepam | | | Use: anxiolytic |
| Ketazolam | 7.5 | 3.2 hrs | 34 - 100 hrs | diazepam N-desmethyldiazepam N-desmethylketazolam | | | Use: anxiolytic<br>Significantly increases latency to REM sleep as compared to baseline, and decreases REM sleep<br>Less sedative than diazepam |
| Lorazepam | 1 | Within 2 hrs (oral) I.M.: 45 - 75 min. | 17 hrs mean (8 - 24 hrs) | lorazepam glucuronide | Metabolite not pharmacologically active<br>Half-life not much affected by age or sex | Cimetidine: no interaction | Use: anxiolytic<br>sedative<br>muscle relaxant<br>manic episode of B.A.D. |

\* Apply to all benzodiazepines except where noted  \*\* Doses are approximate (Alprazolam & Clonazepam are relatively less potent when dealing with anxiety, relatively more when dealing with panic)

*Continued*

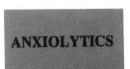

**ANXIOLYTICS**

# A Comparison of the Benzodiazepines (cont'd)

| Drug | Equivalent Dose ** | Peak Plasma Level p.o. | Elimination Half-life | Metabolites (m = main metabolite) | Comments | Clinically Significant Interactions | Clinical Considerations |
|------|------|------|------|------|------|------|------|
| **Lorazepam** (cont'd from pg 37) | | I.V.: 5 - 10 min Subling.: 60 min | | | Clearance reduced in elderly by 22% (1 study) Slow onset of action Give at least twice daily to maintain steady state levels | | Half-life and Vd doubled in patients with cirrhosis Significant anterograde amnesia produced, which doesn't correlate directly to its sedative potency Blood levels fall quickly on discontinuation; withdrawal symptoms appear sooner than with long-acting drugs Decreases stage 1 and time spent in REM; increases stage 2 of sleep |
| **Nitrazepam** | 2.5 | 3 hrs mean (0.5 - 7 hrs) | 29.5 hrs mean (18 - 98 hrs) | No active metabolites | Excreted as amino and acetamide analogues | | Use: sedative Age does not affect clearance, but elderly more sensitive to sedative and depressive effects (not attributed to kinetics) |
| **Oxazepam** | 15 | 2 - 3 hrs | 9 hrs mean (3 - 25 hrs) | Ooxazepam glucuronide | Metabolites not pharmacologically active Half-life and plasma clearance not affected much by age or sex Slow onset of action Give at least twice daily to maintain steady state | Food: little influence on either rate or extent of absorption Cimetidine: no interaction | Use: anxiolytic, sedative, alcoholism treatment, muscle relaxant Can cause withdrawal insomnia Half-life not significantly affected by liver disease Used as "hostility tranquilizer" since can lower aggression levels in patients with a history of belligerence and assault without releasing paradoxical rage responses |
| **Prazepam** | 10 | 2.5 - 6 hrs | 30 - 100 hrs (metabolites) | Desmethyldiazepam (m) Desalkylprazepam 3-hydroxyprazepam Oxazepam | Prazepam inactive; converted to active metabolites | | Use: anxiolytic |

| | | | | | | | |
|---|---|---|---|---|---|---|---|
| **Temazepam** | 10 | Hard gelatin capsule: peaks at 2 1/2 hrs mean | 9 hrs mean mean (3 - 13 hrs) | No active metabolites | 5% excreted as oxazepam in the urine. Plasma concentration too low to detect | | Use: sedative<br>On doses of 30 mg/day or more, 7% of patients reported hangover, morning nausea, headache, drowsiness and vivid dreaming<br>Doesn't suppress REM, but delays first REM period, shifting it towards the latter portion of sleep<br>Decreases sleep stages 3 & 4<br>Rebound insomnia has been reported |
| **Triazolam** | 0.25 | 2 hrs | 2.2 - 4.1 hrs | 7-$\alpha$-hydroxy derivative | Metabolite inactive<br>Negligible accumulation of drug | Desipramine: report of hypothermia with the combination(neither drug causes this effect alone)<br>Potentiation of anorexic effect of desipramine | Use: sedative<br>Although half-life is short, clinical effects have been observed up to 16 hrs after a single dose<br>Decreases stage 1, and increases stage 2 of sleep; significantly increases latency to REM as compared to baseline<br>Rebound insomnia and anxiety reported<br>Anterograde amnesia reported, especially in doses above 0.5 mg daily |
| **Azaspirodecanedione Deriv.**<br>**Buspirone** | | 5 .7 - 1 hr | .9 - 9.4 hrs (parent) | 1-(2-pyrimidyl) pipirazine | Onset of action takes days to weeks<br>Maximum effect seen in 3 - 4 weeks | Does not interact with alcohol<br>No clinically significant interaction reported | Use: anxiolytic<br>Low potential for abuse or dependence<br>No cross-tolerance with benzodiazepines (will not alleviate benzodiazepine withdrawal)<br>No muscle relaxant or anticonvulsant properties<br>Use cautiously in seizure disorder |

\* Apply to all benzodiazepines except where noted

\*\* Doses are approximate

**ANXIOLYTICS**

# MOOD STABILIZERS

**CLASSES**

Lithium Carbonate

Carbamazepine

## Lithium Carbonate

**INDICATIONS**

- Long-term control of manic depressive (bipolar affective) disorder
- Prevention or diminution of the intensity of subsequent episodes of mania and depression
- May potentiate the action of cyclic antidepressants and MAO Inhibitors
- Treatment of acute mania
- Treatment of chronic aggression/antisocial behaviour

**PHARMACOLOGY**

- Exact mechanism of action unknown; postulated that lithium may stabilize catecholamine receptors, and may alter calcium-mediated intracellular functions
- Lithium therapy requires reaching plasma concentrations that are relatively close to the toxic concentration
- Administration of lithium requires 10-14 days before the complete effect is observed, therefore acute mania is usually treated with a neuroleptic; lithium is subsequently added to the treatment regimen

**PHARMACOKINETICS**

- Peak plasma level: 1 1/2 - 2 hrs (slow release preparation = 4 hrs)
- Half-life: 8 - 35 hrs; once daily dosing preferred
- Therapeutic Plasma level: 0.4 - 1.2 mmol/L (patients in an acute manic episode appear to have an increased tolerance to lithium)
- Excreted primarily by the kidney; therefore, adequate renal function is essential in order to avoid lithium accumulation and intoxication

**ADVERSE EFFECTS**

a) These coincide with peaks of serum lithium concentration and are probably due to rapid absorption of the lithium ion. Most disappear after a few weeks:

G.I. irritation (nausea, abdominal pain, loose stools), muscular weakness, restlessness, slurred speech, blurred vision, dazed feeling, vertigo

b) These may persist for long periods, but are reversible and disappear when lithium is withdrawn:

Fine tremor of the hand (propranolol may be of benefit), fatigue, non-toxic goiters, polyuria, polydipsia, edema, weight gain

c) Miscellaneous - occur occasionally:

Headache, dryness and thinning of hair, leg ulcers, skin rash, acne, exacerbation of psoriasis, pruritis, metallic taste, transient hyper-glycemia, anaemia, leukopenia, leukocytosis, albuminuria, arrhythmias, ECG changes, toxic confusional states, choreoathetotic movements, seizures

d) Long-term effects: Renal damage, hypothyroidism, hyperparathyroidism

## PRECAUTIONS

- Good kidney function, adequate salt and fluid intake are essential
- Decreased sodium (Na⁺, salt) intake or excessive loss (due to vomiting, diarrhea, use of diuretics, etc) causes increased lithium retention, possibly leading to toxicity.
  ☞ DO NOT GIVE to patients on salt-free diets
- Use cautiously and in reduced dosage in the elderly as the ability to excrete lithium decreases with age
- Some researchers suggest that concurrent ECT may increase the possibility of developing cerebral toxicity to lithium
- Avoid abrupt withdrawal, if possible; 50% rate of manic recurrence among previously stable patients reported

## CONTRAINDICATIONS

- Brain damage
- Renal disease
- Cardiovascular disease
- Severe debilitation
- Conditions requiring low sodium intake

## TOXICITY

### Mild

- At lithium levels of 1.5-2 mmol/L
- Develop gradually over several days
- Side effects such as ataxia, coarse tremor, confusion, diarrhea, drowsiness, fasciculation and slurred speech may occur
  <u>Treatment</u>: Stop lithium

### Moderate to Severe

- At lithium levels in excess of 2 mmol/L
- Severe poisoning may result in coma with hyperreflexia, muscle tremor, hyperextension of the limbs, pulse irregularities, hypertension or hypotension, ECG changes, peripheral circulatory failure and epileptic seizures
- Deaths have been reported; when serum lithium level exceeds 4 mmol/L the prognosis is poor

<u>Treatment</u>:
Symptomatic: Restore fluid and electrolyte balance, correct sodium depletion
Blood lithium concentration may be reduced by forced alkaline diuresis or by prolonged peritoneal dialysis or hemodialysis
Excretion may be facilitated by I.V. urea, sodium bicarbonate, acetazolamide or aminophylline
Convulsions may be controlled by a short-acting barbiturate (thiopental sodium)

## NURSING IMPLICATIONS

- Accurate observation and assessment of patient's behaviour before and after lithium therapy is initiated is important
- Be alert for, observe and report any signs of side effects, or symptoms of toxicity
- Check fluid intake and output. Adjust fluid and salt ingestion to compensate if excessive loss occurs through vomiting or diarrhea
- May give lithium with meals to avoid G.I. disturbances
- Withhold lithium on mornings when blood is drawn for lithium leve

## USE IN PREGNANCY

- Avoid in pregnancy (especially first trimester); preponderance of cardiovascular malformations seen

### Breast Milk

- Present in breast milk at a concentration of 30-100% of mother's serum. Discourage breast feeding

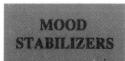

**MOOD STABILIZERS**

# Lithium Carbonate (cont'd)

## PATIENT INSTRUCTIONS

- The patient and family should be educated regarding the drug's effects and toxicities
- Watch for signs of early toxicity (diarrhea, vomiting, drowsiness, muscular weakness, ataxia). Withhold the dose, call the doctor immediately
- Expect transient nausea, polyuria, thirst and discomfort during the first few days
- Expect a lag of 1-3 weeks before the full beneficial effects of the drug are noticed
- Maintain adequate salt and fluid intake. Do not go on any special diets without consulting the physician
- Avoid driving a car or operating hazardous machinery until response to the drug is determined
- Carry an identification/instruction card with toxicity and emergency information, or wear a medic-alert bracelet
- Get lithium levels done regularly and have an outpatient follow-up of thyroid and renal functions every 12 months. Do not take lithium dose the morning of the blood test

## BIOCHEMICAL WORK-UP

At beginning of treatment:

(1)   ECG
(2)   serum electrolytes
(3)   Hb, Hct, WBC and differential, ESR
(4)   BUN, creatinine

(5)   T4, T3, resin uptake, TSH
(6)   calcium
(7)   parathormone

## DRUG INTERACTIONS

Repeat tests (3) to (5) every 6 months and at every admission; (6) every two years; (7) after 5 years, thereafter yearly

| Class | Example | Interaction Effects |
|---|---|---|
| Anaesthetic | Ketamine | Increased lithium toxicity due to sodium depletion |
| Angiotensin-converting enzyme inhibitor | Captopril | Increased lithium toxicity due to sodium depletion |
| Antibiotics | Ampicillin, tetracycline, spectinomycin | Increased lithium effect and toxicity due to decreased renal clearance of lithium |
| Anticonvulsants | Carbamazepine, phenytoin | Increased neurotoxicity of both drugs<br>Synergistic mood stabilizing effect with carbamazepine |
| Antidepressants | Cyclic and MAOI's | Synergistic antidepressant effect |
| Antihypertensives | Amiloride, spironolactone, thiazides, triamterene<br>Acetazolamide, mannitol, urea | Increased lithium effects and toxicity due to decreased renal clearance of lithium<br>Increased renal excretion of lithium, decreasing its effect |
| Bronchodilators | Aminophylline, theophylline | Increased renal excretion of lithium, decreasing its effect |
| L-tryptophan | | Increased plasma level and increased efficacy of lithium |
| NSAIDS | Ibuprofen, indomethacin, naproxen | Increased lithium effect and toxicity due to decreased renal clearance of lithium |
| Neuroleptics | | Decreased neuroleptic blood level<br>Increased neurotoxicity at therapeutic doses |

# Carbamazepine

**INDICATIONS**

- Anticonvulsant, with particular efficacy in temporal lobe and limbic region seizure disorders
- Paroxysmal pain syndromes, e.g. trigeminal neuralgia
- Treatment of dystonic disorders in children
- Diabetes insipidus
- Management of affective disorders, particularly in bipolar patients who are either rapid cyclers or lithium non-responders.  Effective in acute mania and in prophylaxis (55-76% response)
- Control of violent outbursts, assaultive behaviour; used alone or in combination with lithium, neuroleptics or ß-blockers
- May work adjunctively with neuroleptics to improve negative symptoms of schizophrenia
- Some improvement in patients with panic attacks and EEG abnormalities
- Alcohol withdrawal

**PHARMACOLOGY**

- Anticonvulsant activity mediated through a "peripheral" type benzodiazepine receptor
- Effective in inhibiting seizures kindled from repeated stimulation of limbic structures
- GABA-agonist activity

**PHARMACOKINETICS**

- Structurally related to tricyclic antidepressants
- Peak levels occur 2 - 6 hours after dosage; maximum blood levels are reached in 2 - 4 days
- 75% bound to plasma proteins
- Half-life is between 25 - 35 hrs after acute administration and 15 - 20 hrs after chronic use. As carbamazepine stimulates its own metabolism, dose adjustment may be required after a few weeks
- Begin at 200 mg daily in divided doses and increase progressively until attain serum levels of 17 - 50 umol/L
  Serum level should be measured at trough (i.e. the last dose is taken 12 hours before level determination

**ADVERSE EFFECTS**

- Can be minimized by initiating treatment at a low dosage, building dose up gradually and having more frequent dosing intervals
- Those seen at the initial phase of therapy include:

  dizziness, drowsiness, ataxia, blurred vision, diplopia, headache, tremors, dry mouth, nausea, chills, fever

- For other common adverse effects refer to chapter on antidepressants
- Haematologic effects (aplastic anaemia, transitory leukopenia, eosinophilia, thrombocytopenia, purpura and agranulocytosis) are sometimes seen and demand immediate cessation of drug treatment.  Mild degree of white blood cell suppression can occur; stop therapy if levels drop below 3000 white cells/mm$^3$
- Severe dermatological reactions may signify impending blood dyscrasia and may necessitate discontinuation of treatment (3% incidence)
- Hepatocellular and cholestatic jaundice have been reported
- Hyponatremia and water intoxication has been reported

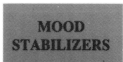

**MOOD STABILIZERS**

# Carbamazepine (cont'd)

**PRECAUTIONS**

- Prior to treatment laboratory investigations should be performed (see below)
- Carbamazepine induces its own hepatic metabolism; therefore, twice-weekly determinations of serum carbamazepine should be done for the first month, weekly for the second month, every other week for the third month, and monthly thereafter
- Because of its anticholinergic action, give cautiously to patients with increased intraocular pressure or urinary retention

**CONTRAINDICATIONS**

- Patients with a history of hepatic or cardiovascular disease or with a blood dyscrasia
- Hypersensitivity to any tricyclic compound

**TOXICITY**

- Occurs if plasma levels above 50 umol/L
- Signs:
  dizziness, ataxia
  drowsiness, stupor
  nausea, vomiting
  agitation, disorientation
  tremor, involuntary movements, opisthotonos, abnormal reflexes
  mydriasis, nystagmus
  flushing, cyanosis and urinary retention
- No known antidote, treat symptomatically

**NURSING IMPLICATIONS**

- Watch out for signs of fever, sore throat and haemorrhage
- Close clinical and laboratory supervision should be maintained (see PRECAUTIONS) throughout treatment to detect signs of possible blood dyscrasias
- A rash may signal incipient blood dyscrasias
- Check for urinary retention and constipation. Increase fluids to lessen constipation
- Warn patient to avoid driving a car or operating hazardous machinery until response to drug has been determined
- Caution patient that alcohol or other depressants will cause an increase in sleepiness, dizziness and lightheadedness

**USE IN PREGNANCY**

- Dosage requirement may drop during pregnancy. Recent report advises of possible teratogenicity in humans

**Breast Milk**

- The American Academy of Pediatrics considers the drug compatible with breast feeding

**LAB INVESTIGATIONS**

Prior to starting therapy the following should be done:
- Complete blood count including platelets and differential
- Liver function tests
- Creatinine
- Serum electrolytes
- EEG
- Some sources recommend complete blood count every 2 weeks for 3 months, then 4 times a year thereafter to monitor for haematopoietic suppression. Transient decreases in white blood count are common. If WBC dips below 3000 mm$^3$, the drug should be stopped.
- Periodic serum electrolytes to check for hyponatremia

| Class | Example | Interaction Effects |
|---|---|---|
| Antibiotics | Erythromycin, troleandomycin | Increased plasma levels of carbamazepine due to reduced clearance (by 5 - 41%) |
| Anticoagulants | | Enhanced metabolism of anticoagulant and impaired hypoprothombinemic response |
| Anticonvulsants | Phenytoin, phenobarbital | Decreased carbamazepine levels as well as anticonvulsant levels, due to enzyme induction |
| Ca-channel blockers | Diltiazem, verapamil | Increased plasma levels of carbamazepine (total carbamazepine increased 46%, free carbamazepine increased 33%) |
| Cimetidine | | Increased carbamazepine levels and increased toxicity |
| Danazol | | Plasma levels of carbamazepine increased by 50 - 100%; half-life is doubled and clearance reduced by half |
| Isoniazid | | Increased plasma level of carbamazepine; clearance reduced by up to 45% |
| Lithium | | Increased neurotoxicity of both drugs; Synergistic mood stabilizing effect; may potentiate antidepressant or antimanic effect |
| Neuroleptics | | Increased neurotoxicity of both drugs at therapeutic doses |
| Oral contraceptives | | Increased metabolism of oral contraceptive may result in decreased contraceptive efficacy |
| Theophylline | | Decreased theophylline level due to enzyme induction by carbamazepine |

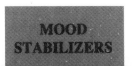

MOOD STABILIZERS

# PARALDEHYDE

Paraldehyde has been available since the late 1800s.

**INDICATIONS**

- Rapid-acting hypnotic (similar to chloral hydrate)
- Treatment of withdrawal delirium and other psychiatric states characterized by extreme agitation. As much as 30 ml orally is given to quiet the patient and induce sleep. By injection, 10 ml is usually sufficient with the occasional need for a further 10 ml after 1 hour
- Emergency treatment of convulsive episodes arising from tetanus, eclampsia, status epilepticus and poisoning by convulsive drugs
- Obstetrical anaesthesia

**DOSING ROUTE**

**Oral**

Sedative:       5 - 10 ml
Hypnotic :    10 - 30 ml
Usual dose range:    3 - 30 ml  maximum of 60 ml within 24 hours

**Rectal**

Retention enema  15 - 30 ml added to 2 volumes of olive oil and given by rectal insertion

**Parenteral: Intramuscular**

Sedative:       5 ml
Hypnotic:     10 ml

**Parenteral: Intravenous infusion**

Sedative:       5 ml     diluted with several volumes of sodium chloride inj.
Hypnotic:     10 ml     diluted as above

**ABSORPTION AND FATE**

- Oral paraldehyde is rapidly absorbed and reaches a maximum concentration after 1/2 hour
- 70 - 80% of the dose is metabolized by the liver; 11 - 28% is exhaled and 0.1 - 2.5% is excreted in the urine

## PRECAUTIONS

- In ordinary therapeutic doses, paraldehyde has little effect on respiration and blood pressure. Large doses cause prolonged unconsciousness with respiratory difficulty, cyanosis, pulmonary edema and acidosis. Hypotension can occur with large doses. Kidney function may be impaired
- Minimum reported lethal dose: 25 mg orally and 12 ml rectally. Fatalities are rare
- Minor side effects include erythematous skin rash and gastric irritation
- Chronic intoxication may cause tolerance and dependence
- Paraldehyde has no analgesic properties and may produce excitement or delirium in the presence of pain
- Use with caution in bronchopulmonary disease and hepatic insufficiency
- Paraldehyde may decompose during storage; use of such material has caused deaths
  DO NOT USE paraldehyde if it smells like acetic acid (vinegar)
- When intravenous paraldehyde is used, the central depression may be preceded by excitement or coughing for a few seconds
- Avoid the use of other sedative drugs (including sedating neuroleptics, benzodiazepines and hypnotics) within 3 hours of using paraldehyde

## CONTRAINDICATIONS

- Orally, in gastroenteritis, especially if ulceration is present
- DO NOT USE rectally in the presence of colitis

## NURSING IMPLICATIONS

- Observe for local irritation of mucous membranes when paraldehyde is administered frequently by mouth or rectum; dilute the drug sufficiently
- To avoid unpleasant taste and irritation of throat and gastric mucosa, the drug can be taken in milk, fruit juices, iced tea or with cracked ice
- Intramuscular injections should be given deep in the buttocks, but care must be taken for nerve damage may occur if injected close to nerve trunks
- Use solution from freshly opened ampoules and within 15 minutes, if the syringe is plastic
  EXPIRY DATES should be checked
- Not more than 5 ml should be injected at any one site; the injection is painful
- Patients should remain on continuous observation for at least 30 minutes and vital signs should be monitored every 15 minutes for 1 hour
Watch for signs of respiratory depression

## DRUG INTERACTIONS

### Disulfiram (Antabuse)

- Paraldehyde is depolymerized to acetaldehyde by the liver; disulfiram impairs the disposition of acetaldehyde by inhibiting acetaldehyde dehydrogenase. Clinical reports of this interaction are lacking, but animal studies and theoretical considerations indicate it may be significant; the use of the two concomitantly should be closely supervised

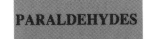

**PARALDEHYDES**

# NEW TREATMENTS OF PSYCHIATRIC DISORDERS

Biochemical theories on the etiology of specific psychiatric disorders have initiated investigations of various drugs/ chemicals that may influence brain neurotransmitters and thereby play a role in the treatment of psychiatric disorders. Several drugs traditionally used to treat medical conditions have been found to be of benefit in ameliorating or preventing symptoms of certain psychiatric disorders. This section presents a summary of some of these drugs and their uses.

## SUMMARY CHART

| | Anxiety | Depression | Sedation | Mania | Schizophrenia | SDAT | Antisocial Behaviour/ Aggression |
|---|---|---|---|---|---|---|---|
| d-Amphetamine | | P | | P | P/S | | |
| Bromocriptine | | + | | C | | | |
| Clonazepam | + | + | | +/S | C/P | | |
| Clonidine | + | | | P/S | + | | |
| Clozapine | | | | | + | | |
| Deanol | | | | | | P | |
| Diltiazem | | | | + | | | |
| Hydergine | | | | | | P | |
| Lecithin | | | | S/P | | P | |
| L-tryptophan | | +/S | + | P/S | | | + |
| Methylene Blue | | P/S | | S | | | |
| Methylphenidate | | +/S | | | | | |
| Methysergide | | | | C | | | |
| Naloxone | | | | P | +/S | P | |
| Nifedipine | | | | | P/S | | |
| Phenytoin | | | | C | + | | + |
| Propranolol | + | | | + | C/S | | + |
| Reserpine | | S | | S | S | | |
| Thyroid Hormones | | S | | C | | | |
| Sodium Valproate | C | | | +/S | C/S | | |
| Verapamil | | | | +/S | P/S | | |
| Mega-Vitamins | | | | | C/S | | |

C = contradictory results     P = potential in proven cat     + = positive     S = suggestive effect

# Adrenergic Agents

*Central stimulating or blocking agents of noradrenergic receptors*

### Clonidine

**A central and peripheral α-adrenergic agonist; acts on presynaptic neurons and inhibits noradrenergic transmission at the synapse**

**ANXIETY**
- Postulated that abnormally high reactivity of brain noradrenergic systems is related to some clinical forms of anxiety
- Dose: 0.15 - 0.5 mg/day
- Of some benefit in generalized anxiety disorder, panic attacks, phobic disorders and obsessive-compulsive disorders
- Psychological symptoms respond better than somatic symptoms
  *(Hoehn-Saric, R. et al., Arch. Gen. Psychiat. 38, 1278-1282, 1981; Jann, M.W. & Kurtz N.M., Clin. Pharmacy 6:12, 947-962, 1987)*

**MANIA**
- Dose: 0.25 - 1.2 mg/day
- Partial but rapid response seen in several patients with mania
- May have a synergistic effect with lithium, carbamazepine and neuroleptics
  *(Bond, W.S., J. Clin. Psychopharm. 6(2), 81-87, 1986)*

**SCHIZOPHRENIA**
- Dose: 0.25 - 0.9 mg/day
- Decrease in psychotic symptoms and gradual improvement in tardive dyskinesia reported
- Response in both positive and negative symptoms seen
- Rebound psychotic symptoms reported on withdrawa
- May relieve neuroleptic-induced akathisia
  *(Freeman, R. et al., Acta Psychiatr. Scand. 65, 35-45, 1982)*

### Propranolol

**A nonspecific beta-blocker with membrane-stabilizing effect and GABA-mimetic activity**

**ANTISOCIAL BEHAVIOUR/ AGGRESSION**
- Dose: 80- 640 mg/day
- Useful in controlling rage, violence, irritability and aggression due to a number of causes
- Positive response reported also with nadolol (40 - 160 mg/day) and pindolol (10 - 60 mg/day), as well as metoprolol
- Rebound rage reactions on drug withdrawal reported; taper dose gradually
  *(Biol. Ther. Psychiat. 9:11, 41-43, 1986; Int. Drug Therapy 20(3), 9-12, 1985)*

**ANXIETY**
- Dose: up to 320 mg/day
- Beneficial for somatic or autonomically mediated symptoms of anxiety (e.g. tremor, palpitations, etc.)
- Positive response also reported with oxprenolol (40 - 240 mg/day), metoprolol (100 mg/day), and atenolol (50 mg/day)
  *(Jefferson, J.W., Arch. Gen. Psychiat. 31, 681-691, 1974)*

**MANIA**
- Dose: up to 2900 mg/day
- Promising results seen in mania
- Depression has been reported
- Clinical usefulness is limited by side effects encountered at the high doses required (encephalopathy is a serious risk at doses > 1000 mg/day)
  *(Jann, M.W. et al., D.I.C.P. 18, 577-589, 1984)*

*Continued*

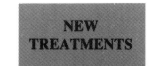

**NEW TREATMENTS**

# Adrenergic Agents (cont'd)

## Propranolol (cont'd)

### SCHIZOPHRENIA

- Dose: up to 5800 mg/day (more commonly: 120-700 mg/day)
- Contradictory results seen
- May be beneficial in acute schizrenia
- Some response seen on negative symptoms
- May increase plasma level of neuroleptic
- Efficacy may be related to treatment of neuroleptic-induced akathisia
- May be useful in controlling aggressive behaviour in schizophrenic patients
  (Lipinski, J.F. et al., J. Clin. Psychopharm 8:6, 409-416, 1988, Biol. Ther. Psychiat. 9(4), 13-14, 1986)

## Thyroid Hormones

**Modulate adrenergic receptor function and permit a given concentration of catecholamines to be more effective**

### DEPRESSION

- Dose: l-thyroxine: 0.1 - 0.5 mg/day
  liothyronine 0.025 mg/day
- Contradictory results seen in refractory depression

- May potentiate effects of antidepressants
- May exacerbate mania
  (Biol. Ther. Psychiat. 9(11), 43-44, 1986)

### MANIA

- Dose: l-thyroxine: 0.3 - 0.5 mg/day
- Reported to alleviate symptoms and increase cycle length in rapid-cycling female patients
  (Stancer, H.C. & Persad, E., Arch. Gen. Psychiat. 39, 311-312, 1982)

# Anticonvulsants

## Clonazepam

**Has GABA-agonist and 5-HT potentiating properties**

### ANXIETY

- Dose: 0.5 - 8 mg/day
- Up to78% of patients reported to experience clinically significant relief from panic disorder
- Useful in agoraphobia with panic attacks; the number of attacks and the intensity of generalized anxiety reported to decrease
  (Rosenbaum, J.F., in New Concepts in Mania and Panic Disorders: Focus on Clonazepam, pp. 35-44 Proc. of Symposium, Vancouver, Can. 1986)

### MANIA

- Dose: 4 - 16 mg/day
- Up to 66% of manic patients exhibiting agitation reported to respond
- May decrease dosage requirements of neuroleptics in both acute treatment and prophylaxis
- Synergistic effect with lithium
- May be useful in preventing antidepressant-induced mania
- 2 case reports of response in rapid-cycling bipolar patients
  (Chouinard, G. in New Concepts in Mania and Panic Disorders: Focus on Clonazepam, pp. 3-14, Proc. of Symposium in Vancouver, Can. 1986)

**DEPRESSION**

- 84% response seen in 25 patients with major depression or bipolar disorder
- 1.5-6 mg/day; rapid onset of activity reported
- Controversial data as to efficacy; may be useful in patients exhibiting agitation
  *(Chouinard, G., in Use of Anticonvulsants in Psychiatry, pp. 43-58, 1988, Oxford Health Care Inc., Clifton N.J.)*

**SCHIZOPHRENIA**

- Dose: up to 3 mg/day
- Found beneficial in 4 patients with atypical psychoses previously unresponsive to neuroleptics
  *(Frykholm, B., Acta. Psychiatr. Scand. 71, 539-542, 1985)*

## Phenytoin

**Stabilizes membranes, has 5-HT potentiating and GABA-agonist properties**

**ANTISOCIAL BEHAVIOUR/ AGGRESSION**

- Dose: 100 - 300 mg/day
- Demonstrated ability to alter emotional lability, impulsivity, irritability and aggression
  *(Lion, J.R., J. Nerv. Ment. Dis. 160(2), 76-82, 1975)*

**MANIA**

- Dose: up to 900 mg/day (no plasma levels done)
- Uncontrolled studies showed improvement in bipolar patients
  *(Jann, M.W. et al., D.I.C.P. 18, 577-589, 1984)*

**SCHIZOPHRENIA**

- Dose: 200 - 300 mg/day
- Beneficial effect on irritability, anger, anxiety and hostility reported in schizophrenic patients
- May be useful in psychotic patients with localized EEG abnormalities
  *(Pinto, A. et al., Compr. Psychiat. 16, 529-536, 1975)*

## Sodium Valproate

**Has anti-kindling effect, anticonvulsant and GABA-ergic activity**

**MANIA**

- Dose: 750 - 3000 mg/day (serum level of 350 - 700 µmol/L)
- Over 50% of patients responded, in a review of 10 studies of over 180 patients with polar or schizoaffective disorder
- Synergistic effect with lithium
- Useful in both acute mania and prophylaxis
- Positive results seen in rapid-cycling patients when used alone or in combination with lithium or a neuroleptic
  *(McElroy, S.L., in Use of Anticonvulsants in Psychiatry, pp. 25-41, 1988, Oxford Health Centre Inc., Clifton N.J.)*

**SCHIZOPHRENIA**

- Inconclusive results (31% response seen in 4 studies)
- Decrease in paranoid ideation and hallucinations reported when used in combination with neuroleptic
  *(Ibid.)*

**ANXIETY**

- One report of improvement in 6 out of 10 patients with panic disorder
- Anxiolytic effects occur at higher doses than anticonvulsant effects
  *(Ibid.)*

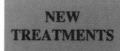
NEW
TREATMENTS

# Calcium Channel Blockers

*Block the reflux of calcium into brain tissue*
*Calcium has wide-ranging effects on the synthesis and release of neurotransmitters, as well as on receptor sensitivity*

### Diltiazem

**MANIA**
- Dose: up to 360 mg/day
- Promising results seen when used together with neuroleptic
  *(Caillard, V., Neuropsychobiol. 14:1, 23-26, 1985)*

### Nifedipine

**SCHIZOPHRENIA**
- Dose: up to 60 mg/day
- Possible effects on negative symptoms when used with neuroleptic
  *(Kramer. M.S. et al., J Clin Psychopharm 7:3, 195-196, 1987)*

### Verapamil

**MANIA**
- Dose: 160 - 320 mg/day
- Useful adjunctive drug in combination with lithium or a neuroleptic
- Used in acute treatment and in prophylaxis
- May prevent antidepressant-induced switches into mania.
  *(Gitlin, M.J., J. Clin. Psychopharm: 4(6), 341-343, 1984; Giannini, A.J. et al., Am. J. Psychiatry 141(12), 1602-1603, 1984)*

**SCHIZOPHRENIA**
- Doses of 160 mg/day
- Some benefits reported in combination with neuroleptic treatment
- Possible effect on negative symptoms
  *(Taurjiman, S.V. et al., Psychopharm. Bull. 23, 227-229, 1987)*

# Cholinergic Agents

*Increase the activity of acetylcholine*

## Lecithin

**MANIA**
- Dose: 15 - 30 g/day
- Response in hallucinations, delusions and affective symptoms
- Depression has been reported
  *(Schreier, H.A., Am. J. Psychiat. 139, 108-110, 1982)*

- Promising results reported when combined with lithium or a neuroleptic
- Stabilized rapid-cycling mood disorder in one patient

**SDAT**
- Dose: up to 24 g/day

  *(Barbeau, A., Le J. Canadien des Sciences Neurol. 5(1), 157-160, 1978)*

- Little improvement in functioning or cognition, but did lessen depression, irritability and anxiety

# Dopaminolytic Agents

*Decrease transmission of dopamine, or block dopaminergic receptors*

## Bromocriptine

**Acts on presynaptic autoreceptors and inhibits dopaminergic transmission at the synapse**
**Acts as a dopamine receptor agonist at high doses and a dopamine receptor antagonist at doses below 40 mg/day**

**DEPRESSION**
- Dose: up to 60 mg/day
  *(Waehrens, J. & Gerlach, J., J. Affect. Dis. 3, 193-202, 1981)*

- Results comparative to imipramine in treatment of depression

**MANIA**
- Dose: 7.5 - 15 mg/day
  *(Jann, M.W. et al., D.I.C.P. 18, 577-589, 1984)*

- Contradictory results seen in manic patients resistant to usual treatments

## d-Amphetamine

**Blocks release and re-uptake of dopamine and norepinephrine**

**DEPRESSION**
- Dose: 5 - 20 mg/day
- Useful in medically or surgically ill patients who meet the criteria for major depression
  *(Currents 6:5, 5-10, 1987)*

- Potentiates cyclic antidepressants
- Response may predict positive treatment with imipramine or desipramine

**MANIA**
- Dose: up to 15 mg/day
- Temporary improvement in mania noted
- Low doses more effective than high doses, as the latter can produce manic behaviour
  *(Brown, W.A. & Mueller, B., Am. J. Psychiat. 136:2, 230-231, 1979)*

*Continued*

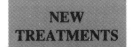
NEW TREATMENTS

# Dopaminolytic Agents (cont'd)

## d-Amphetamine *(cont'd)*

**SCHIZOPHRENIA**
- Dose: up to 50 mg/day
- Improvement reported in mood, concentration, and anxiety in 32 of 48 patients also receiving neuroleptics
- Some improvement in negative symptoms in combination with neuroleptics
  *(Cesarec, Z. & Nyman, A.K., Acta Psychiatr. Scand. 71, 523-528, 1985)*

## Methylphenidate

**DEPRESSION**
- Dose: 10-20 mg/day
- Potentiate cyclic antidepressants in treatment-resistant patients
- Useful in medically or surgically ill patients who meet the criteria for major depression
  *(Askinazi, C. et al , J.Clin. Psychiat. 47, 467-469, 1986; Biol.Ther. Psychiat. 10(9), 35-38, 1987*
- May be useful in withdrawn or apathetic elderly patients
- Females tend to respond better than males

# Narcotic Antagonists

## Naloxone

**Postulated to produce an anti-hallucinatory effect by displacing endorphins from opiate receptors**

**MANIA**
- Dose: 0.4 - 20 mg I.V.
- Short-lived benefit seen in mania
  *(Janowsky, D.S. et al., Lancet 2, 320, 1978)*

**SCHIZOPHRENIA**
- Dose: 0.4 - 28.5 mg I.V.
- Conflicting results reported
- Relief in hallucinations and symptomatic improvement seen in patients within 24-48 hours
- May potentiate neuroleptic activity
  *(Pickar, D. et al., Arch. Gen. Psychiat. 39, 313-319, 1982)*

**SDAT**
- Dose: 1 - 10 mg I.V.
- Temporary positive effect on cognition seen
  *(Reisberg, B. et al., N.E.J.M. 308, 721-722, 1983)*

# Serotonergic Agents

*Elevate the levels of serotonin*

## L-Tryptophan

**A serotonin precursor**

**ANTISOCIAL BEHAVIOUR/ AGGRESSION**

- Dose: 4 - 8 g/day
- Has shown positive results in decreasing aggression in normal as well as in schizophrenic subjects
(*Young, S.N., 'The Clinical Psychopharmacology of Tryptophan' in Nutrition and the Brain, Vol. 7, eds. R.J. Wurtman & J.J. Wurtman, 1986*)

**DEPRESSION**

- Suggested that serotonergic activity is decreased in a subgroup of depressed patients
- Dose: up to 16 g/day (in divided doses)
- Positive results seen in some patients when used alone in depression
- Potentiate effects of cyclic antidepressants
- Some benefits in prophylaxis
(*Byerley, W.F. et al., J. Clin Psychopharm. 7(3),127-137, 1987*)

**MANIA**

- Dose: up to 12 g/day
- Conflicting results seen when used alone or in combination with neuroleptics
- May potentiate effects of lithium in acute mania or prophylaxis of bipolar affective disorder
(*Pakes, G.E., D.I.C.P. 13, 391-396, 1979*)

**SEDATIVE HYPNOTIC**

- Dose: 1 - 5 g/day. Best administered 30-45 minutes before bedtime
- Doses up to 5 g daily increase the amount of sleep without distorting usual stages of sleep (as above)
- Improvement reported after several days of administration; efficacy does not diminish over time
(*Biol. Ther. Psychiat. 11:4, 13-16, 1988*)

---

## Methysergide

**Antiserotonin agent**

**MANIA**

- Dose: 3 - 6 mg/day
- Conflicting results reported
- Inhibits excessive psychomotor activity and drive and normalizes sleep
- Depression reported
(*Jann, M.W. et al., D.I.C.P. 18:577-589, 1984*)

---

## Reserpine

**DEPRESSION**

- Dose: 2.5 - 10 mg/day
- Potentiates effects of antidepressants in patients with treatment-resistant depression
- Response seen in 42 of 50 patients (reports from a number of studies)
(*Biol. Ther. Psychiat. 20(5), 17-18, 1985*)

**MANIA**

- Dose: 0.25 - 1 mg/day
- Useful in combination with lithium; lithium may protect against reserpine-induced depression
(*Bacher, N.M. & Lewis, H.A., Am. J. Psychiat. 136, 811-814, 1981*)

**SCHIZOPHRENIA**

- Reported useful in approximately 50% of chronic schizophrenics when given in combination with neuroleptic
- Useful in patients with agitation, paranoia and affective intensity
(*Berland, J.L., J. Clin. Psychopharm. 6(3), 180-184, 1986*)

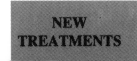

**NEW TREATMENTS**

# Miscellaneous

## Clozapine

**"Atypical" neuroleptic: more selective for $D_1$-receptors; selective for limbic system; minimal effect on prolactin**

### SCHIZOPHRENIA

- Dose: 25-900 mg/day (twice as potent as chlorpromazine)
- Antipsychotic activity similar to that of the standard neuroleptics; may be useful in patients refractory to other treatments
- Minimal extrapyramidal effects; may alleviate tardive dyskinesia; useful for psychoses in patients with Parkinson's Disease
- Commonly produces sedation, hypersalivation, hypotension and hyperthermia
- Caution: up to 7% incidence of agranulocytosis and up to 9% risk of seizures reported
  *(Bablenis, E. et al., D.I.C.P. 23:2, 109-115, 1989)*

## Hydergine

**Cerebral vasodilator containing ergot**

### SDAT

- Dose: ergot up to 12 mg/day
- Improvement seen in behavioural and psychological measures (e.g. mental alertness, orientation, locomotion, etc., but not in cognitive functions)
- May yield some benefit particularly for patients with milder degrees of impairment
- Possible antidepressant action, since ergot alkaloids inhibit norepinephrine re-uptake *in vitro*
  *(Gulevich, G., in Psychopharmacology, p. 464, J.D. Barchas et al. (Eds.), 1977)*

## Methylene Blue

### DEPRESSION

- Dose: up to 200 mg/day
- Useful when combined with lithium in prophylaxis
  *(Naylor, G.J. et al., Biol. Psychiat. 21, 915-920, 1986)*

### MANIA

- Dose: up to 200 mg/day
- Possible synergistic effect when combined with lithium (as above)

## Megavitamins

### SCHIZOPHRENIA

- Dose of niacin or nicotinamide: up to 3 g/day
- A study by the Canadian Mental Health Association in 1970, trying to duplicate results reported by Dr. A. Hoffer,
  found that niacin alone had little benefit in schizophrenia
  *(Ban, T.A. & Lehmann, H.E., Can. J. Psychiat. 20, 103-112, 1975; Hoffer, A., Drug Therapy 7, 79-85, 1977)*
- Reports that ascorbic acid in doses up to 8g/day may antagonize dopamine neurotransmission and potentiate activity of the neuroleptic
  (may antagonize the metabolism of the neuroleptic)
  *(Biol. Ther. Psychiat. 11:1, 2-3, 1988)*

# GLOSSARY

**AGRANULOCYTOSIS** — Reduction of white blood cells to very low levels

**AKATHISIA** — Inability to relax, compulsion to change position, motor restlessness; usually drug induced (common with neuroleptics)

**AKINESIA** — Absence of voluntary muscle reaction, lack of movement

**AMENORRHEA** — Absence of menstruation

**ANOREXIA** — Lack or loss of appetite for food

**ANTICHOLINERGIC** — Blocking the passage of impulses through the vagus nerve, thus inhibiting secretion of gastric juices, reducing the motility of the G.I tract and enhancing the action of antacids

Causes dry mouth, blurred vision, constipation, etc.

**ANTIEMETIC** — Helps prevent nausea and vomiting

**AREFLEXIA** — No reflexes

**ARRHYTHMIA** — Any variation of the normal rhythm (usually of the heart beat)

**ARTERIOSCLEROSIS** — Hardening and degeneration of the arteries due to fibrous tissue formation

**ARTHRALGIA** — Pain in the joints

**ASTASIA ABASIA** — Inability to stand or walk

**ATARACTIC** — Causing calmness of mind

**ATAXIA** — Muscle incoordination, especially the inability to coordinate voluntary muscular action

**ATHEROSCLEROSIS** — Degeneration of the walls of the arteries due to fatty deposits

**AUTONOMIC** — The part of the nervous system that is functionally independent of thought control (involuntary)

**B.A.D.** — Bipolar affective disorder (manic-depressive illness)

**BRADYCARDIA** — Abnormally slow heart beat

**BRAIN STEM RETICULAR FORMATION** — Nerve network of part of the brain (deals with alertness)

**CHOREIFORM** — Purposeless, uncontrolled sinuous movements, jerking

**CHOREOATHETOID** — Slow, repeated, involuntary sinuous movements or twitching of muscles

**CHRONIC BRAIN SYNDROME** — Irreversible damage to brain cells

**CNS** — Central nervous system

**CNS DEPRESSION** — Drowsiness, ataxia, incoordination, slowing of respiration which in severe cases may lead to coma and death

**CORTEX** — The external layer (superficial gray matter) of the brain

**CORYZA** — "Head cold," acute catarrhal inflammation of nasal mucosa

**DERMATITIS** — Inflammation of the skin

**DIAPHORESIS** — Perspiration

**DYSARTHRIA** — Impaired, difficult speech

**DYSPHAGIA** — Difficulty in swallowing

**DYSKINESIA** — Loss or impairment of the power of voluntary movement leading to abnormal movements, i.e. twitching, grimacing

**DYSTONIC REACTIONS (DYSTONIAS)** — Disordered muscle tone leading to spasms

**E.C.G.** — Electrocardiogram (tracing electrical activity of the heart muscle)

**E.C.T.** — Electroconvulsive therapy, "shock therapy"

**E.E.G.** — Electroencephalogram (tracing of electrical activity of the brain)

**EDEMA** — Swelling of body tissues due to accumulation of tissue fluid

**EMESIS** — Vomiting

**ENDOCRINE** — A gland that secretes internally, a ductless gland

**ENDOGENOUS DEPRESSION** — Depression from within. In DSM III, called Major Affective Disorder

**ENZYME** — Organic compound that acts upon specific fluids, tissues or chemicals in the body to facilitate chemical action

**ENURESIS** — Involuntary discharge of urine

**EPIGASTRIC** — Referring to the upper middle region of the abdomen

**EXACERBATION** — Increase in severity of symptoms or disease

**EXTRAPYRAMIDAL** — Refers to certain nuclei of the brain close to the pyramidal tract

**EXTRAPYRAMIDAL DYSFUNCTION** — Causes Parkinsonian-like effects and/or impaired muscle tone

**FASCICULATION** — Twitching

**GABA** — Gamma-amino butyric acid; an inhibitory neurotransmitter

**GALACTORRHEA** — Excretion of milk from breasts

**GLAUCOMA** — A condition of increased pressure within the eye

**GYNECOMASTIA** — Increase in breast size in males

**HYPEREXCITEMENT** — Over-excitement

**HYPERREFLEXIA** — Increased action of the reflexes

**HYPERKINETIC** — Abnormal increase in activity

**HYPERTENSION** — High blood pressure

**HYPNOTIC** — Inducing sleep

**HYPOTENSION** — Low blood pressure

**INDURATION** — Area of hardened tissue

**JAUNDICE** — Yellow appearance of skin caused by excess of bile pigment

**KINDLING** — Eleptogenesis caused by adaptive changes in neurons due to repeated electrical discharges

**LDH** — Lactic dehydrogenase (an enzyme)

**LIBIDO** — Psychic drive or energy usually associated with sexual instinct

**LIMBIC SYSTEM** — A system of brain structures common to the brains of all mammals (deals with emotions)

**LOCOMOTOR ACTIVITY** — Movement

**M.A.O.** — Monoamine oxidase (an enzyme)

**MANIC DEPRESSIVE PSYCHOSIS** — Conspicuous mood swings ranging from normal to elation or depression, or alternating of the two. In DSM-III, called Bipolar Affective Disorder

**MIOSIS** — Constricted pupils

**MYALGIA** — Tenderness or pain in muscles, muscular rheumatism

**MYDRIASIS** — Dilated pupils

**NARCOLEPSY** — A condition marked by an uncontrollable desire to sleep

**NYSTAGMUS** — Involuntary movement of the eyeball or abnormal movement on testing

**OCULOGYRIC CRISIS** — Rolling up of the eyes and the inability to focus

**OCCIPITAL** — In the back part of the head

**ORTHOSTATIC HYPOTENSION** — Faintness caused by suddenly standing erect (leading to a drop in blood pressure)

**PARKINSONISM** — A condition marked by masklike facial appearance, tremor, change in gait and posture. A common side effect of neuroleptic drugs

**PERIORAL** — In the mouth area

**PERIPHERAL NEUROPATHY** — Pathological changes in the peripheral nervous system

**PHOTOPHOBIA** — Sensitivity of the eyes to light

**PHOTOSENSITIVITY** — Easily sunburned

**PISA SYNDROME** — A condition where an individual leans to one side

**POSTURAL HYPOTENSION** — Lowered blood pressure caused by a change in position

**PROSTATIC HYPERTROPHY** — Enlargement of the prostate gland

**PSYCHOSIS** — A major mental disorder of organic or emotional origin in which there is a departure from normal patterns of thinking, feeling and acting; commonly characterized by loss of contact with reality

**PSYCHOMOTOR EXCITEMENT** — Physical and emotional overactivity

**PSYCHOMOTOR RETARDATION** — A generalized retardation of physical and emotional reactions

**PSYCHONEUROSIS** — Emotional maladaptations usually due to unresolved unconscious conflicts

**PYLORIC** — Referring to the lower opening of the stomach

**RABBIT SYNDROME** — Perioral tremor, particularly of the lower lip

**SCHIZOPHRENIA** — A severe emotional disorder of psychotic depth characterized by a retreat from reality with delusions and hallucinations

**SDAT** — Senile dementia Alzheimer's type

**SEDATIVE** — Producing calming of activity or excitement

**SIALORRHEA** — Excessive flow of saliva

**SYNCOPE** — A sudden loss of strength or fainting

**TACHYCARDIA** — Abnormally rapid heart rate

**TARDIVE DYSKINESIA** — Persistent dyskinetic movements that appear late in therapy, often when the neuroleptic dose is decreased or discontinued. Consists of smacking and licking of lips, sucking or chewing movements, grotesque grimacing, choreoathetoid movements of the extremities, etc.

**THERAPEUTIC INDEX** — Ratio of median lethal dose of a drug to its median effective dose: i.e, therapeutic index = $\dfrac{\text{lethal dose 50\%}}{\text{effective dose 50\%}}$

**TINNITUS** — A noise in the ears (ringing, buzzing or roaring)

**TORTICOLLIS** — Spasm on one side of the neck causing the head to twist or tilt

**TRACKING** — A reaction in which the medication leaves the original injection site and moves to another

**TRISMUS** — Severe spasm of the muscles of the jaw resembling tetanus (lock jaw)

**VASOCONSTRICTOR** — Causing narrowing of the blood vessels

# REFERENCES AND SUGGESTED READINGS

## Antidepressants

Ananth, J. (1983). Choosing the right antidepressant. *The Psychology Journal of the University of Ottawa, 8(1)*, 20-26.

APA Task Force on Laboratory Tests in Psychiatry (1987). The dexamethasone suppression test: An overview of its current status in psychiatry. *American Journal of Psychiatry, 144(10)*, 1253-1262.

Bernstein, J.G., & Bernstein, D.B. (1987). Psychotropic-related weight gain. *Drug Therapy, 17(4)*, 109-119.

Briggs, G.G., Freeman, R.K., & Yaffe, S.J. (1983). *Drugs in pregnancy and lactation* (2nd ed.). Williams and Wilkins.

Coccaro, E.F., & Siever, L.J. (1985). Second generation antidepressants: A comparative review. *Journal of Clinical Pharmacology, 25*, 241-260.

Davidson, J. (1983). When and how to use a monoamine oxidase inhibitor. *Drug Therapy, 13(1)*, 197-202.

Editorial (1985). Adverse reactions to MAOI's. *Biological Therapies in Psychiatry, 8(1)*, Jan.

Gerner, R.H. (1983). Systematic treatment approach to depression and treatment-resistant depression. *Psychiatry Annals, 13(1)*, January.

Perry, P.J., Alexander, B., & Liskow, B.I. (1988). *Psychotropic drug handbook* (5th ed.). Harvey Whitney.

Quitkin, F. *et al.* (1979). Monoamine oxidase inhibitors. *Archives of General Psychiatry, 36*, 749-760.

Rosenbaum, J. F., & Pollack, M.H. (1987). Managing antidepressant side effects (interview). *Currents, 6(11)*, 5-13.

Sullivan, E.A., & Shulman, K.I. (1984). Diet and monoamine oxidase inhibitors: A re-examination. *Canadian Journal of Psychiatry, 29(8)*, 707-711.

Swartz, C.M., & Sherman, A. (1984). The treatment of tricyclic antidepressant overdose with repeated charcoal. *Journal of Clinical Psychopharmacology, 4 (6)*, 336-340.

Zisook, S. (1984). Side effects of isocarboxazid. *Journal of Clinical Psychiatry, 45(7)*, 53-58, July.

Simeon, J.G. (1989). Pediatric Psychopharmacology. *Canadian Journal of Psychiatry, 34(2)*, 115-122, March.

## Neuroleptics

Barchas, J.D. *et al.* (Eds.) (1977). *Psychopharmacology: From theory to practice.* New York: Oxford.

Chouinard, G. *et al.* (1986). A controlled clinical trial of flupirilene, a long-acting injectable neuroleptic, in schizophrenic patients with acute exacerbation. *Journal of Clinical Psychopharmacology, 6(1)*, 21-26.

Cohen, B.M. *et al.* (1986). Plasma levels of neuroleptic in patients receiving depot fluphenazine. *Journal of Clinical Psychopharmacology, 5(6)*, 328-332.

Editorial (1980). How high the neuroleptics. *Biological Therapies in Psychiatry, 3*, 10, October.

Jann, M.W. *et al.* (1985). Clinical pharmacokinetics of the depot antipsychotics. *Clinical Pharmacokinetics, 10*, 315-333.

Jeffries, J.J. (1987). The use of neuroleptics. In E. Persad & V. Rakoff (Eds.), *Use of drugs in psychiatry: A handbook* (pp. 1-21). Toronto: Hans Huber.

Mason, A.S., & Granacher, R.P. (1980). *Clinical Handbook of Antipsychotic Drug Therapy.* New York: Brunner Mazel.

## Antiparkinsonian Agents

Donlon, P.T. (1973). The therapeutic use of diazepam for akathisia. *Psychosomatics, 14,* 222-225.

Wong, J. (1985). Antipsychotic induced extrapyramidal side effect. *Canadian Pharmaceutical Journal, 118(9),* 15 January.

## Anxiolytics

Committee on the Review of Medicines (1980). Systematic Review of the Benzodiazepines. *British Medical Journal,* March 29, 910-912.

Cooper, A.J. (1983). Benzodiazepine update: A guide to rational prescribing. *Modern Medicine, 38,* 209-218.

Devenyi, P., & Saunders, S.J. (1986). *Physician's handbook for medical management of alcohol and drug related problems.* Toronto: Addiction Research Foundation.

Editorial (1980). New perspectives in benzodiazepine therapy. *Arzneimittel Forschung, Drug Research, 30(1),* 851-916.

Greenblatt, D.J. (1983). Pharmacokinetic properties of benzodiazepine hypnotics. *Journal of Clinical Psychopharmacology 3(2),* 129-139.

Sellers, E.M. (1978). Clinical pharmacology and therapeutics of benzodiazepines. *Canadian Medical Association Journal, 118,* 1523-1538.

Solomon, F. (1979). Sleeping pills, insomnia and medical practice. *New England Journal of Medicine, 300 (14),* 803-808.

## Mood Stabilizers

Editorial (1982). Carbamazepine, acute and prophylactic effects in manic and depressive illness: An update. *International Drug Therapy Newsletter, 17(2,3),* 5-9.

Jann, M.W. *et al.* (1984). Alternative drug therapies for mania: A literature review. *Drug Intelligence & Clinical Pharmacology, 18,* 577-589.

Jefferson, J.W. *et al.* (1983). *Lithium encyclopedia for clinical practice.* American Psychiatric Press.

Post, R.M. (1988). Effectiveness of carbamazepine in the treatment of bipolar affective disorder. In *Use of anticonvulsants in psychiatry,* eds. McElroy, S.L. & Harrison, G.P., Oxford Health Care Inc.

## New Treatments of Psychiatric Disorders

Galizia, V. (1984). Pharmacotherapy of memory loss in the geriatric patient. *Drug Intelligence & Clinical Pharmacology, 18,* 784-791.

Jann, M.W. *et al.* (1984). Alternative drug therapies for mania: A literature review. *Drug Intelligence & Clinical Pharmacology, 18,* 577-589.

Lerer, B. (1985). Alternative therapies for bipolar disorder. *Journal of Clinical Psychiatry, 46,* 309-316.

McElroy, S.L. & Harrison, G.P. (1988). Use of Anticonvulsants in Psychiatry. Oxford Health Care Inc., Clifton, N.J.

**Hans Huber Publishers**

Toronto • Lewiston, N.Y. • Bern • Göttingen • Stuttgart

serving the medical and social science communities
for more than three generations.

---

## ORDER FORM

**NO POSTAGE CHARGE WITH PREPAYMENT**
Discounts with bulk orders of 10 copies or more:
Enquire for details

Please send me ———— copy (ies) of

### Clinical Handbook of Psychotropic Drugs
(US $19.95/CAN $24.95)

☐ Check in the amount of ———————— enclosed
☐ Bill me
☐ Put my name on your mailing list
☐ Send information on new titles in the following area(s):

———————————————————————

☐ Send complete catalogue

Name: ————————————————

Address: ——————————————

Make cheque payable to and send order to:
HOGREFE & HUBER Publishers

CANADA
12-14 Bruce Park Ave.
Toronto, Ontario  M4P 2S3
☎  (416) 482-6339
Fax: (416) 484-4200

U. S. A.
P. O. Box 51
Lewiston, N.Y.  14092
☎  (716) 282-1610
☎  (800) 228-3746

---

**Hans Huber Publishers**

Toronto • Lewiston, N.Y. • Bern • Göttingen • Stuttgart

serving the medical and social science communities
for more than three generations.

---

## ORDER FORM

**NO POSTAGE CHARGE WITH PREPAYMENT**
Discounts with bulk orders of 10 copies or more:
Enquire for details

Please send me ———— copy (ies) of

### Clinical Handbook of Psychotropic Drugs
(US $19.95/CAN $24.95)

☐ Check in the amount of ———————— enclosed
☐ Bill me
☐ Put my name on your mailing list
☐ Send information on new titles in the following area(s):

———————————————————————

☐ Send complete catalogue

Name: ————————————————

Address: ——————————————

Make cheque payable to and send order to:
HOGREFE & HUBER Publishers

CANADA
12-14 Bruce Park Ave.
Toronto, Ontario  M4P 2S3
☎  (416) 482-6339
Fax: (416) 484-4200

U. S. A.
P. O. Box 51
Lewiston, N.Y.  14092
☎  (716) 282-1610
☎  (800) 228-3746